WOMAN DESIRED,
WOMAN DESIRING

D1599074

WOMAN DESIRED, WOMAN DESIRING

Danièle Flaumenbaum

AEON

Aeon Books
PO Box 76401
London W5 9RG

British Library Cataloguing in Publication Data

A C.I.P. for this book is available from the British Library

ISBN-13: 978-1-91280-764-2

Typeset by Medlar Publishing Solutions Pvt Ltd, India

Printed in Great Britain

www.aeonbooks.co.uk

CONTENTS

INTRODUCTION   ix

CHAPTER ONE
We love men like we love our mothers   1
   The first object of love   2
   Loving like a child   2
   The woman and the mother in us   4
   Why do we regress when we love?   6
   Maternal love is not sexual   6

CHAPTER TWO
The dynamic of sexual anatomy   9
   The circulation of sexual energy   9
   The role of the uterus in sexual pleasure   13
   The clitoris, the hymen and the vagina   14
   The uterus, the fallopian tubes and the ovaries 17
   Hormonal control   19
   The lesser pelvis, the hips and the perineum   20
   Breasts and breastfeeding   23
   Changes and transformations in a woman's body   23
   Setting sexual energy in motion   25

CHAPTER THREE

The barrier of fire: recurrent disorders   29

  Acute ailments, recurrent ailments   29

  Looking for the origin   31

  Fire in the genitals: blocked sexuality   33

  Chinese medicine   36

  Disrupting the repetition   37

  Making love   38

  Teaching our genitals about pleasure   40

  The life force that inhabits us   42

CHAPTER FOUR

How little girls construct their sexuality and how

  daughters come undone when their mothers die   45

  Expecting a little girl   45

  At birth, the child becomes the magnetic catalyst   47

  The power of names and surnames   48

  Breast-feeding   50

  Building the baby girl's sexuality   52

  The dyad stage   55

  Wanting to know the true story   57

  Finding self-recognition   59

  The father's role and the difference between sexes   60

  Telling a little girl that later her genitals

    will welcome a man's   64

  Parental intimacy   65

  "But where was I before?"   67

  The bottomless pit: falling into depression   69

  Quest for meaning and renewal   72

CHAPTER FIVE

The gynaecological family tree   75

  Painful menstruation   75

  "Phantom" disorders   81

  Premenstrual syndrome   82

Gynaecological ailments and their origins   83
Symptoms generated by family line disorders   85
Sterility and infertility   86
Unwanted pregnancies   86
The importance of knowing one's genealogy   87
The effects of building a genosociogram   89
Care   92

CHAPTER SIX

Desire   95
Inherited social and cultural burdens   96
First change: women think (1945)   97
Second change: birth control (1965)   97
Third change: sexual liberation?   98
Parental fulfilment   100
Continued ignorance about sexuality   100
Desire: the energy that makes the encounter possible   101
When desire is inhibited   102
The body is not invaginated   105
How to break the cycle of transgenerational
    repetition   106
The starting point of a man's sexual desire is the
    genitals, while a woman's is in her heart,
    between her two breasts   109
Woman and their desire: floating heads   111
So, what is desire?   112

CHAPTER SEVEN

What is making love?   113
Courtship displays   114
Creating a shared space: foreplay and
    the encounter between the genitals   114
Fondling the breasts   117
Fixation on the clitoris   118
Desired, but also desiring   119

Benefitting from what we do not have 121
The co-penetration of the genitals 122
Creating the phallus 123
Feeling the uterus and maintaining the fire 123
Being fully present to oneself and
    to the other at the same time 125
Finding words again 125
Pathways of sexual energy 126
Completeness and surpassing oneself 127
Projecting oneself into the other's body 127
Jouissance: sexual joy 128
What is an orgasm? 129
Coming down after making love 132

ACKNOWLEDGEMENT 133

INDEX 135

INTRODUCTION

I was born during the Second World War, the third of three daughters. My sisters were eleven- and fifteen-years older than me. My parents, Polish Jews in hiding within the free zone in the south of France, had heard that pregnant women and those who had children under the age of one would not be deported to the concentration camps. My father had lost his mother when he was three years old and was worried about saving his wife and daughters. My mother, who had just lost her own mother whom she loved unconditionally, was absorbed mourning her loss. So, I was born to save my mother and sisters, as the ray of sunshine that could bring life back to human folly. On top of all that, my maternal grandmother, whom I never met and whose name I bear, was a midwife. It was only natural then that I should perpetuate her by becoming a gynaecologist.

Although I loved natural science, languages and travelling, medical school was baffling. I had a hard time during my medical studies. The curriculum was too dense. I could not digest so much information in so little time. We had to know everything, and I felt my life was passing me by. I made friends including the man who would become my first husband. We were activists, fighting for a practice of medicine in which patients were considered not just as numbers, but as individuals with emotions, feelings and unique backgrounds.

Providing medical care to women meant helping them to respect themselves: they had a brain connected to a body, and I believed both should get along even though brains and bodies do not seem to function in the same way. Women of my generation had seen our parents suffer from isolation, each one shut off into his or her own world, incapable of speaking to and understanding the other. In my generation, women would have a freer life, as alter egos to men; we would become their companions. I did not anticipate the personal work required for this transformation of social roles.

During the first twelve years of my gynaecological practice, in which I divorced, did a first "round" of psychoanalysis, and met the father of my children, it was Chinese medicine and training in acupuncture that opened me to the idea of energy and introduced me to Chinese sexology. The ancient Chinese did not only describe pathways taken by sexual energy. They also explained how sexual activity was necessary for illness prevention, mental health and longevity. Their explanations satisfied the woman gynaecologist who was looking for a way to link the body with the mind.

The majority of women I met in my practice suffered from not being able to experience their sexuality in the way they wanted: feeling comfortable with their sensations, adjusting and exchanging them with those of their partner and, as a result, knowing the restorative benefits that come from shared love.

I began my career in 1971. At the time like nearly all the women of my generation, despite difficulties in my own personal life, I believed that the pill would automatically guarantee a fulfilling sex life. It seemed obvious that the pleasure of being a woman would automatically follow on from the pleasure of being a modern mother who had, only recently, seen her right to work recognized.

We had all suffered from the straitjacket imposed on our parents and grandparents that forbade and inhibited sexuality. We were going to be able to live a freer life. We felt lucky. And yet today, two generations after this liberation, even though our outlook on life has changed radically, women who come to see me—be they twenty, thirty, forty or fifty years old—are still caught in the grip of sexual difficulties. Relations between men and women continue to be a source of incomprehension, fatigue and drama.

Why do sexuality and sexual fulfilment, now accepted as social norms, continue to be so difficult to translate into real life? Why do our bodies not know how to feel desire or experience the pleasure of the sexual encounter to the fullest when the body has the capacity and inclination to do so?

Lifting the moral ban should be all it takes. Yet, wanting and being permitted to enjoy one's sexuality are not enough to feel at ease. The intimate does not necessarily follow the social because like all human functions and values that involve the body but are not its preserve, carnal love is the outcome of early transmissions we receive during infancy, information which moulds us and imprints our cells.

Little girls will only dream about becoming 'mummy' if their own mother was a happy one. Girls must be able to grow up knowing that the sexuality they will experience when they are older will give them both pleasure and strength. "If the mother is herself proud to be a woman and happy to have a daughter, everything is in order for the child, allowing her to invest her femininity and her genitals in a positive way," wrote French psychoanalyst Françoise Dolto (1). Otherwise, these same little girls will continue to be modelled on the old pattern, social and family propriety dictating that not only should they not show anything, or say anything about the pleasure of sexuality, but that sexuality itself was to be banished. This silence and incoherent self-expression blocks spontaneity and is at the root of the dissatisfaction, fear, confusion and shame experienced by many girls during sexual maturation. When young girls become women, they always carry with them the baggage they inherit from their families.

I myself was destined to become a happy mother with a profession, but I was never encouraged to become a sexual woman. The magic and strength of sex had not existed at all in my family. Its place in adult life was not handed down as a value. Quite to the contrary, my genitals did not exist or rather, even while being part of my morphology, they remained an enigma. They were nameless, and I did not know how they worked.

For women, making love is not only about giving herself over and surrendering to the man she loves. It is also about knowing how to welcome him and receive him inside, both into her mind and heart but also her genitals. For those who choose to embark on the journey, sex can lead to the discovery of a greater self and partner. For Hadrien, Marguerite Yourcenar's hero, this journey progresses from the love of a body to the love of a person (2). For others, this journey will bring them from the love of a person to the love of a body.

Sexuality is the privilege of adulthood that one discovers as a teenager. It evolves progressively and needs to adjust at each stage of life. A journey involves separating from and leaving what is known in order to open up to the unknown. With sex, the setting changes, bringing new landscapes and atmospheres with novel colours, scents, music and languages. It is a matter of taking the time to appreciate and integrate all these splendours so as to become stronger, richer and increasingly oneself. The more the pleasure of this journey becomes part of life, the more beneficial it can be. For that pleasure to exist, however, and to be able to appreciate it when it is present, we have to know the codes and what is at stake. Otherwise, we may miss out on this marvel, unable to find our way or paralyzed with fear by the new experience. Another risk—and one that is often the case—is to fail to take the trip.

Saying yes to integrating sexuality into one's life means saying yes to the journey and to discoveries made along the way. Both my life as a woman and my experience as a gynaecologist have shown me the extent to which, even today, women are still not readied for the journey of encounter between the sexes: they continue to be caught in a web of false beliefs and of ignorance.

Until my generation—the post-war generation—this journey was harshly judged, even forbidden. The ban disappeared with the advent of contraception in the mid-1960s. It is now socially accepted that women, like men, can live out their sexuality. But they still do not know how to imagine sex with a joyful attitude. They consent but remain completely inert. The pains and ailments that translate tragedies inherited from females in their family, catch up with women and stand in the way of their own desire. In the 1960s, French singer Georges Brassens said that "95% of women are bored when they screw." This figure accurately reflected the reality of the time. Today, I would say that the figure is barely less than 85%.

Most women consider themselves open to loving the other's body and their own, but as we will see, they often remain closed without knowing it. This closure is invisible and cannot be felt. These women certainly desire to embark on sexuality's journey. They dream of it, but they remain paralyzed by a sexual education burdened with ignorance and taboo. They remain stuck on the threshold or in the vestibule, waiting to be "carried away" or initiated.

Our sexuality takes root within the emotional and affective climate of the family into which we are born. The way that family considers sexuality—the idea they have of it and the place they assign to it in their lives—literally models our behaviour and lays the foundation for how we communicate with others. It constitutes our "primary structuration" that creates our foundations and the conditions for what Françoise Dolto calls our "secure base" (3).

Yet, without even realizing it, these women are still prisoners of the fear and taboos in which their mothers, aunts and grand-mothers were confined. They shaped themselves by identifying with these women, and so they are made like them. Their mothers could not release them from this confinement, because they did not know they themselves were shut in.

As long as their mothers remained "girls," daughters too remain "girls."

Dissatisfaction, conscious or unconscious frustration, sadness, fatigue, rows, anger: men and women do not know how to talk to each other, nor how to take the time to listen. It's always the other's fault. Unable to step back or to conceptualize the differences in the way men and women function, they withdraw, usually snapping shut like oysters, the men retracting like snails.

Welcome and reception are at the essence of the feminine dynamic. When these notions are ignored, they both hinder and deflect the benefits of erotic encounter. Allowing the other's sexual energy to enter one's body brings about regeneration, revitalization and a feeling of wholeness. This encounter of the flesh is not just a matter of trading feminine and masculine sexual energy. It is an alchemy that bolsters those energies enabling both partners to enjoy the benefits of what each does not have, thereby transcending the self. This enjoyment is a passage into another dimension of the real, causing us to grow through the encounter with newness and proximity to the mystery of life. It is where sexuality and sacrality meet.

My mother and her generation could not hand down this sexuality of pleasure, because they did not know it existed. My generation promoted an "anything goes" attitude, giving rise to permissiveness but not a lived experience available to pass on. Women today should accept that they have not been constructed to experience this pleasure and therefore must acknowledge the need to learn.

Such was my experience as a woman. It allowed me to discover that I was not built any differently from the patients I saw. Like them, I identified with old models. It took me years before I could hear, accept and integrate the idea that I did not behave like a "woman," even though I was already a mother. The shock came as a blow.

I was going on forty and the man I loved, the father of my children, whose undertakings I supported and whom I respected, kept telling me he did not have a "woman" in his life.

I could not understand what he was saying. He did not know how to explain further, and I was unable to deeply listen to what he meant. It was during lovemaking when he put all his ardour into it one night that I opened up like never before. I suddenly felt his energy invade my body and flow through me: I was welcoming him in. I could not get over it. It felt like I was a new woman, someone else. I had undergone a mutation. Then I understood. That was the pleasure, the orgasm, the climaxing sexual joy—"*jouissance*" (4)—he had been talking about.

Once this sexual openness established itself, my life was never the same again. I no longer saw the world in the same way, a door had opened, a curtain had been lifted. I had landed on a planet where everything was vast, and this new birth of myself expanded me, gave me greater stature. Not only could I unfold my limbs and stand up straighter as if I had spent my previous life in a dollhouse, I also felt lighter, having jettisoned attachments to the past that had blocked my spontaneity. I became more flexible and stronger, because I was receiving new energies. Making love became the capacity to welcome and receive the energies of the man I loved inside me. I discovered the value of his genitals and in turn made him feel his power, confirming him as a man. Until then, I had been able to show him my love by giving, supporting and taking care of him. I had been able to give myself over to him, but only "on the surface." He obsessed my heart and mind, but I did not yet know how to welcome him sexually by taking him and his energy inside of myself.

Since then, this revitalizing sexuality has become an integral part of my life. I understood that to keep it alive required giving it time, that I had to learn to prepare myself, and make myself ready for an encounter with my partner. I was amazed by the vitality that this new life gave me and just could not understand why I never had the keys before. There was nothing disgusting, vulgar or complicated about it. It was, on the contrary, disconcertingly simple. All the nonsense, lunacy and wickedness in my education had led to my being ashamed of my genitals. These "dirty parts," now restituted, became worthy and honourable. I had lost a chastity belt without even knowing that I had one. My genitals became part of my life. I felt whole—quite simply normal.

Sexuality is among the most difficult of human activities, because it demands that the most intimate part of ourselves be in contact with someone else's most private parts. Setting up sexual communication is not magic. It entails a lot of effort, a reshaping of oneself. It is a task that has to be taken seriously for the encounter to happen at all and for it to develop over time.

Notes

1. Françoise Dolto, *La Sexualité féminine* (Paris: Gallimard, 1996), p. 154.
2. Marguerite Yourcenar, *Mémoires d'Hadrien* (Paris: Gallimard, 1977).
3. See Françoise Dolto, *Le Sentiment de soi. Aux sources de l'image du corps* (Paris: Gallimard, 1997).
4. In French, the word "*jouissance*" is used here, a word that has no exact equivalent in English. In French, as powerfully captured in the text at this point, *jouissance* (from 'joy') includes

pleasures of the soul, spirit and body that one fully tastes, which of course include orgasm. However, orgasm(e) has a mechanistic connotation in both languages, a more narrowly corporeal flavour. For readability, the term "sexual joy" has been used throughout this translation. However, to designate key moments, "jouissance" has been adapted as it has been by certain philosophical and psychoanalytic works in English. [Translator]

CHAPTER ONE

We love men like we love our mothers

"It was natural for me to merge completely with the man I loved," said Therese. "For me, that's what it meant to be a woman who loved her man. I felt so happy married to my husband. I sat on his lap with his arms around me, and he would tell me stories and kiss me. He was my Prince Charming. He made me laugh. His love nourished my body. I knew so little about sexuality that I thought melting into him in this way was to make love. I came alive only through my husband. I held my breath when I heard him climbing the stairs. In my heart I was always fulfilled, even before we touched. I scrubbed him in the bath. I was totally happy, but my genitals were not, nor were his either. We saw ourselves as responsible adults, but in fact we were just children. Honestly, without realizing it, we found our happiness in the kind of love that a mother and child share—and our roles were interchangeable. I never felt sexual pleasure when he penetrated me. The example I followed in love was the tenderness I had shared with my mother."

Falling in love reconnects us powerfully to the emotions and attachment we experienced during our first love story: the one we all had with our mother. This original memory is sometimes so strong that it prevents a woman from recognizing the sexual identity of her lover as different. She confuses her love for him with the bond she has with her mother. So long as we love a man the way we loved our mothers, we cannot become sexual women. That is why a woman can love a man without loving his genitals. She loves him, but she has no desire to be penetrated by him. That is how love can become a misunderstanding, a problem or a trap.

The first object of love

When life begins, our mother is our whole world, the world in which our being was constructed. Before we know how to separate ourselves from our mothers, before we can say the word "I," she is our "everything." We inserted ourselves inside of her, creating a body in common. Passively, we are nurtured by her. When we abandon ourselves to the man we love, we relive the memory of this time of oneness when, as infants, we lived entirely inside our mother's physical, energetic and psychic space. As soon as a man becomes our "everything," as soon as we commit ourselves to a shared life with him because we are intimately happy to have found him, we are taken back to when we were not separate from our mother. By its very nature the carnal relationship returns us to that condition (1). Our memory is imprinted with it. Love is the reliving of that feeling which every child, boy or girl, has known with their mother, during the period of utter dependence that begins at conception. In love, we "recontact" the condition that allowed us to come to life. Our mother's role was to carry us, to nourish us, to provide for all our vital needs. The man we love will now take up the place in us that our mother once occupied. We are once more completely dependent.

Loving like a child

You and your mother shared a single body. You occupied the same psychic space and needed no words to understand each other, because at that phase of life communication is by nature telepathic (2). If this symbiosis is reproduced exactly with a man and takes up the whole space, a woman no longer needs to be confronted with the wish to be supported and the pleasure of supporting a man. As Therese put it so well, she melted altogether into the man she loved so that she could rediscover the joy of the fusion she had known with her mother. For her, love still meant sameness and likeness.

When you can give yourself entirely to the man you love, when you abandon yourself to him, it reawakens the total confidence of a baby curled up inside its mother's womb. But at the same time, in wanting him to be the same as you, you do away with the difference between the sexes. For example, to want the man we love to understand us and to fulfil us without needing to say a word, harks back to the time when the baby girl did not yet speak in words. To make herself understood she expressed herself through intonations, calls and facial expressions largely modelled on those of her mother, enabling her to communicate. The magic of being understood without needing words, the pleasure of it, derives from that early phase of life. Wanting the man we love to understand us without having to talk to him in words means relying on him to the extent of expecting him to understand us like a mother would. "But I'm not inside your head! You're secretly asking me for the moon but I'm a sun!" cries a man to his beloved during a spat.

When they form a couple, lovers recreate a shared space that re-enacts the duo that constructed them. But unless you see the sexual relationship as a journey that goes beyond the limits of the embrace experienced with mother, the man and woman will remain confined in tenderness. They will warm each other's body and heart and comfort each other's soul without understanding why their genitals are not invited to the dance. They love each other, but they don't know they still function like a child. They are happy to be together, they abandon themselves to each other, but, because they only know how to recreate or repair the embrace shared with their mothers, they retreat into a state of symbiosis and are no longer engaged in the dynamic construction of themselves as adults.

To attach oneself to a man we love with love and tenderness alone inevitably creates dependence. The resulting inertia means that the woman not only loses her initiative but also her desire for sexual penetration. The arrow of time is hence reversed. She recedes into an infantile eroticism, which albeit uninhibited, playful and delicious remains forever on the surface.

> "I know nothing about psychoanalysis, but it makes sense that I might confuse my husband with my father. Anyway, that's something I can imagine. But confusing my husband with my mother: I would never have thought of that," a patient told me.

The psychoanalytic concepts that have spread through our culture for some time now focus on how a woman searches for a man to love who resembles her beloved father, or the father she would have wanted. This is true, but it applies to a little girl's life from the age of three. Before that, in the first three years of life, a little girl constructs her identity through the affective embrace in which she and her mother are locked. That is why the men we choose are more likely to separate us from our mothers than to resemble our fathers. But that does not stop us from also loving them the way we loved our mothers!

The woman and the mother in us

> "When I had my child," said my patient Françoise, "I couldn't distinguish between myself as a mother and

myself as a woman. I didn't realize that they weren't one and the same. No woman had ever told me that the thoughts, feelings and emotions of a woman are not identical to those of a mother. For me, the woman and the mother had always been one and the same. I was sure that to be a mother you necessarily had to be a woman, or rather that you became a woman when you bore a child. I told myself that the reason our mothers had not been happy as women was only because they were overburdened with maternal tasks. I had never met a woman who saw sexuality as a regenerative force that renewed her personal energy. As a motherly woman, I confidently waited for my sexuality to blossom. I thought all I had to do was make a few positive adjustments to what I was raised to believe. I never realized I would have to question those beliefs. In my family, sexuality was not explicitly forbidden; it just didn't exist. Only now am I discovering that sexual pleasure does me good, gives me confidence, makes me live, drives me forward."

For Françoise, sexuality was not forbidden but its adult form was poorly understood. The lack of a sexual education did not stop her from falling in love, any more than it prevented her from giving birth. Falling in love opens the heart, but that openness does not necessarily extend to the genitals. It opens a woman to caresses, kisses and tenderness. It awakens feelings and emotions of confidence and of sharing just like those of an infant who is carried, washed, changed and caressed by her mother. We use the same terms of endearment: sweetheart, baby, darling. These words make us feel good and reassure us. But if we remain at that stage instead of asserting ourselves as adults, we will regress without realizing or understanding why sexuality is not really part of our life, or, rather, why we do not experience it fully.

Why do we regress when we love?

Each step in life that moves us forward creates an emotion that throws us off balance. Regression is a natural process that takes us back to something familiar, an emotional context that we already know, and so restores our confidence. We can get back on our feet, gather our strength to take ourselves in hand and find stability again. Regression makes it possible to find a stable foundation within ourself, restoring our secure base from which to get moving again. It does us good; it heals us. When we fall in love, regression takes us back to our infantile sensuality and softness. Returning to the baby's state of total confidence in his/her mother, we are reassured and can open up to the prospect of constructing a new world with our partner. For men and women alike, it is because we had a mother who gave us love and security that we are able to give ourselves to somebody else.

Confident, unstinting, unconditional love is not being called into question here. Falling in love with a man reawakens the power of love that we felt for our parents, and this is what gives romantic love its intensity. But it is important to realize that maternal love is not enough, neither for the fulfilment of our own adult life nor to ensure a properly functioning long term relationship. Adult love includes experiencing the joyful intensity of one's genitals and the celebration of the coming together of the sexes. It is something that is learned.

Maternal love is not sexual

"I was not unloved. I lacked instruction," said Corinne, a woman of my own age. "Out of ignorance I remained maternal with the men I loved. I loved them as if I were their mother. As I grew older, I realized that, in a couple, maternal love leads sooner or later to abuse and painful separations. Each claims to be right, and both get hurt."

Living under the same roof recreates the space you intimately shared with your mother. So, becoming the helper, assistant and comforter of the man you love lends itself to another kind of confusion. The woman who loves her man like she loved her mother will also love him as if he were her child. If she herself had an abusive or intrusive mother, or a lost and absent mother, she will, sooner or later, follow suit and reproduce the pattern she is familiar with. She will become abusive and invasive, or absent—or both!

The great danger in loving maternally is that you believe you know best for someone else. Either a woman begins treating her beloved like a child ("Don't come home too late! Don't catch cold! Be careful!"), or else she knows better than him how he should behave. Without realizing it, Corinne began to act like this with her first husband: "Since we were 'as one', I thought I knew everything about him. I knew what he ought to do without needing any input from him. That was how my mother behaved with my father. I didn't realize he couldn't stand this attitude and that it made him want to run. I found I had become much more intrusive than I would have dreamed possible, I who was so sweet and respectful …."

This kind of invasive behaviour blocks desire and makes a man withdraw into himself like a snail retracting into its shell. People cannot desire each other unless they are separate entities. You can be your partner's helper, assistant and comforter—that is part of love. But that love must allow both partners to breathe and live as they wish.

Mistaking your beloved for your mother or mistaking him for your child amounts to the same thing; both have the effect of banishing sexual desire. For a couple to spread its wings, be propelled forward and mature, a man and a woman must appreciate each other by cherishing their differences.

It is not a woman's maternal qualities that put the couple at risk. It is how those qualities tend to invade the couple's entire shared life that annihilates sexuality. For the maternal to remain generous, it needs to be energized by the feminine.

"In my family," Corinne continued, "we venerated our mother and respected our father, but there was no such thing as men or women. You didn't become a man or a woman. Our parents were forever the sons or daughters of their own parents. They were 'asexual'." In a world like this, where "everyone was everything to everyone else," how could a little girl get her bearings? In being happy as a mother, and in giving her child a father who is happy to be a father, a mother shows her daughter the way to her own future motherhood. In being happy in her womanhood, sharing and experiencing sexual pleasure with the man she loves, a mother opens up for her daughter the prospect of becoming a woman ready to take on her share of pleasure and creativity in her sex life.

Maternal love is not sexual, and for a child's sake it must not be so. As adults, however, we need to make room for and vivify our anatomy so as to renew ourselves and develop. Our genitals are a source of life whose function is to make us independent by separating us from our family and to propel us forward so that we become ourselves. Unless we use our sexuality to fortify ourselves, a part of us will always be "the little girl," who is unhappy and dissatisfied because she is incomplete. It would be as if a man's love could never equal what you experienced, or yearned to experience, with your mother.

Notes

1. See Didier Dumas, *Et si nous n'avions toujours rien compris à la sexualité?* (Paris: Albin Michel, 2004).
2. This is the time of the mother–child dyad, when the child constructs herself by duplicating the mental structures of those who take care of her. It is all conflated: me–my mummy, me–my daddy, me–my little brother, me–my nanny. See Chapter 4, on the construction of the little girl.

CHAPTER TWO

The dynamic of sexual anatomy

The circulation of sexual energy

"Today," Catherine told me, "I'm here for an anatomy lesson. I'm fed up with having cystitis" (1). Although Catherine had been seeing me for some time, I had not realized that she couldn't visualize her body or that she didn't know how it functioned. So, using a dummy and diagrams, I gave Catherine an anatomy lesson. I showed her the pelvic girdle and the organs contained in that cavity, which is the main support of our bodies. It is sealed at the bottom by a strong and complex muscle, the perineum, known as "the muscle of the ancestors" in Chinese.

On a cross-sectional diagram I showed her the parts that were causing her discomfort—the bladder and its excretory duct, the urethra—and their relationships to the vagina, the uterus and the clitoris. I showed her how the urethra is right next to the vagina, just below the clitoris, with the bladder at the front of the uterus, and I explained: "Sexual arousal, which is a fiery form of life energy, necessarily encroaches on the urinary tract. When this energy can circulate freely, when the woman is secure and confident enough to give herself over to the pleasure of the encounter, this energy, spontaneously receptive and welcoming, moves naturally through the vagina to the uterus.

When the energy is thrown off course, through a lack of requisite education, the natural pathway of the energy stagnates or turns in on itself and causes infection in the urinary system." Catherine agreed, "I've noticed that my cystitis often acts up after I've seen my mother or when I experience the desire to make love as shameful. It was at its worst when I actually committed to Christian. I spent our entire honeymoon trip wearing diapers so to speak!"

With cystitis, all the sexual energy is concentrated outside the sex organs. Instead of being able to move through the vagina and the uterus, it goes up into the urethra and the bladder. It is no surprise that Catherine felt so bad: her symptoms separated her from her love bond. Without a doubt, she loved Christian and this disjunction was not about her loving feelings but about the underlying emotions. It happened systematically in a specific emotional context. Going to see her mother, or inversely, separating herself from her mother by marrying Christian, re-connects her with the mother–daughter energy that emotionally destabilizes her. Catherine then regresses to be a little girl. She no longer even knows that she has a vagina. She becomes a little girl once more, scared she will "pee in her pants," spending her honeymoon continually running to the bathroom instead of making love with the husband she adores.

Catherine's cystitis stopped her from experiencing her sexuality. It prevents her from being a woman who allows herself to experience sexual pleasure to the full. Of course, this was not a conscious choice. But her cystitis made it clear that she had never moved beyond her original energetic construction, handed down to her by her mother and the other women in her family, for whom pleasure did not exist. Catherine lacked neither desire nor sexual energy: if she were devoid of sexual energy, she would have felt nothing. The energy was there, but it was displaced and inverted. It had turned against her in the urinary system. It burned Catherine; it hurt her and stopped her from venturing out into her life as a sexual woman. With Catherine, I realized that I should be giving more anatomy lessons.

When I was Catherine's age, I too needed to know how my body worked. But my knowledge of descriptive anatomy from my studies was static and could not effectively support me in my life as a woman. I knew how I was made, how I ovulated, how my body changed during pregnancy. I knew about giving birth. But I did not know how my genitals could come alive and be part of me, nor how they functioned with a partner in achieving pleasure. I was taught anatomy for mothers.

When I studied acupuncture, I learned how the circulation of life energy in me animated my physical body. I came to see my anatomy as a precious tool, alive and dynamic. I learned to be aware of the circulating flow of energy, to explore it, to identify and understand the internal functions of my body and to mentally get in touch with the parts that are unwell in order to restore or establish proper energy circulation. This was quite a challenge, and still is today.

Love and feelings are not enough to bring our genitals to life. Loving a man does not do away with the taboos and inhibitions stored up since infancy, or even before birth, that stand in the way. When it comes to pleasure and sexual fulfilment, our disastrous legacy from our mothers, who were incapable of explaining to us what it means to be a woman (2), remains with us. Women today are still uninformed about their genitals. They are still afraid of a man's genitals; fearful of submitting to them, they do not dare to see them as an object of pleasure to be discovered and honoured, even though, anatomically speaking, male and female genitals are clearly made to fit together and this fit brings us benefits and celebrates life.

Chinese traditional medicine and its erotic dimension taught me how the sexual body functions, showing me the womanliness of my own body as well as what happens in the lovers' exchange, "the art of the bedchamber," as the books call it (3). The Taoist civilization of ancient China saw sexuality as essential to health, both physical and mental. Sexual energy contained and generated in the ovaries and in the testicles is one of our great reservoirs of vitality. If we know how to be in touch with this energy, we can learn to revitalize ourselves so the strength we need to live can flourish, ensuring our health, clarifying our mind, keeping away illness. The basic principle of Chinese medicine is that "without sexuality, the spirit cannot flourish" (4). For me, it was a revelation that sexual energy has such a central place in health. It confirmed what I had sensed intuitively, but above all it gave me a tool for enhancing my own and other women's lives.

Taoism, as far as I know, is one of the rare traditions that has so precisely described the processes of sexual encounter and the paths taken by sexual energy. When we make love, sexual energy circulates through the usual energy networks that maintain our daily life, but it also taps into vascular networks of "extraordinary energy" pertaining to the urogenital system, which relate to a far older construction, one that goes back to the embryonic phase (5), and contributes to balancing and regenerating our entire being.

In this way we consolidate, reshape, and strengthen our original structure. This reaffirms our existential base, giving strength, calm and security by restoring lovers to the "genius of their genitals" (6). If the anatomy and functioning of our genitals remain a mystery then sexual union is blocked, and, as a patient put it to me, sexuality will always have an uncertain element. Sexual desire surges unpredictably. We know exchanging sexual energy gives us pleasure, but we do not know how to cultivate it and even less how to take it further. Talking about our genitals not as reproductive organs but as a vibrant part of ourselves, liberates their function to bring pleasure and fulfilment, making us happy to be women.

The role of the uterus in sexual pleasure

Carnal communication implies openness and receptiveness to the other and to the other's sexual energy. Because feminine sexual energies are both attractive and receiving (attracting into oneself), and masculine sexual energies are emissive (propelling oneself outwards), the alchemy of sex comes from the union of these two forces, which, as the Chinese say, "co-penetrate" (7) in lovemaking.

A woman's principal organ for receiving sexual energy is not her vagina but her uterus. The uterus plays a dual role. It is the womb where a new being is created and shaped. But for a woman it is also the place of evolving self-creation, which the Chinese consider vital to the spirit's development. The uterus is the "alchemical cauldron," the chamber of resonance where feminine and masculine forces meet and become one. Knowing how to receive a man's sexual power into one's uterus brings about true re-creation, both of the self and the other. To achieve this, a woman's body must allow masculine energy to go through her cervix into her uterus. But, as we have seen with cystitis, poor knowledge of this process and lack of sexual education mean that for many women the energy remains blocked inside the vagina, causing pain there.

When our genitals are alive, they vibrate. Pleasure consists of feeling the vibrations created by sexual intercourse. If the wiring is good, there is communication between the two, similar to how an electric current circulates from a positive pole to a negative pole. To feel this vibration is to perceive how your partner's energy unites with your own, inside you; to feel the interpenetration of feminine and masculine forces coming together and finding the right balance to resonate together. This resonance allows the sexual energy of each partner to unite at the same frequency, harmonizing the energy outside and inside and vastly increasing pleasure, up to its highest peak: orgasm.

Since energy is made to circulate, if it is not blocked, the united sexual forces can continue on their way, flooding the inside of the body, moving to and fro between one partner and the other, nourishing the organs, straightening the spinal column and rising upwards through the brain to the orifices of the nose, mouth, eyes and ears. When they reach the head, sexual breaths dissolve blockages and clear the mind. One feels more complete, reunited, revitalized. The love partners feel for one another is reconfirmed; they are restored and enriched.

The clitoris, the hymen and the vagina

Continuing our journey through the feminine anatomy, we discover that the genitals are largely inside the body, with only the vulva visible. Viewed from the front, the vulva forms a longitudinal crevice bordered by the labia major. Spreading open the labia major, we see the crevice is circumscribed by the labia minor, which come together at the top as a hood for the clitoris and at the bottom, just before the anus, at the fibrous central core of the perineum. The vulva is also called the mouth of the vagina, since the labia minor surrounding the vaginal opening is made of a tissue that looks and functions like the tissue making up our mouth.

For a woman's genitals to be welcoming, they have to be involved and engaged. Otherwise they are dry, closed, and insensitive, causing pain to both partners. With arousal, they become warm and damp. To achieve this, a whole range of glands, such as Bartholin's glands that line the mucous membranes, are called into play to secrete their lubricating substance. This is why one hears that women "get wet."

The **clitoris** is an erectile bud also called a "glans," like the head of a man's penis. It is located under the pubic bone, hooded by the coming together of the labia minor. Made of a spongy tissue that engorges with blood when there is arousal, its size can change dramatically. It is very sensitive, a focal spot for female sexual pleasure. The pleasure generated by caressing the clitoris helps lubricate the vulva but does not always bring about the desire to be penetrated. Stimulating the clitoris manually, along with a scenario of images or words, leads to orgasmic pleasure that brings harmony to the entire body. This pleasure is so intense that many women fixate on it, sometimes to the point of believing the clitoris provides the greatest pleasure a woman can possibly experience.

It is wrong to say that a woman is either clitoral or vaginal. These are two different kinds of orgasm; they do not have the same effect, but they are complementary. Clitoral orgasm harmonizes a woman's own energy, making her feel suddenly more alive. It is an orgasm that puts us in contact with ourselves and feeds our sense of being. The sexual joy that comes from penetration by a man's penis is produced by the meeting of masculine and feminine energy. This union regenerates both partners. It is the joy of being simultaneously with oneself and with the other. Yet, to be capable of being with the other, one must first be capable of being with oneself. Otherwise, we merge into our partner, no longer able to perceive that he is different. If we fail to understand him as different, we cannot perceive him as a complement to us.

"I am no longer ashamed of my clitoral orgasms. It's really wonderful to stop being ashamed of a part of my own body," Elisabeth told me, both comforted and surprised after we talked about it. What had she been ashamed of? She had been ashamed of experiencing pleasure by touching herself. She thought it was improper, that one ought not to resort to that kind of orgasm. It was a transgression. It was a pleasure she had no right to pursue or to experience since nobody had ever told her about it.

We discover clitoral orgasm in childhood, by solitary masturbation or with a girlfriend or boyfriend during early sexual exploration, or else with a lover at the beginning of our sexual life. In Elisabeth's case, her shame arose not only because she had received no sexual education as a little girl but also because, both as a child and then as a woman, her upbringing cordoned her off from sexuality by shrouding it in silence. I was the first woman in her life with whom she dared to speak of it, even though she was already a young grandmother.

The **hymen** is the frontier between a woman's external and internal sexual organs. It is made of reinforced flesh that forms a ring around the vagina that varies in tightness, keeping it partly closed. Contrary to popular belief, it is not a closed membrane. If it were, menstrual blood would be unable to flow out before a woman first has sex. The hymen's elasticity and extensibility allow some women to lose their virginity without tearing the skin or bleeding. It depends on how you allow your body to participate in the event. Losing your virginity, being deflowered, means leaving childhood behind, going through the portal to womanhood. It is a fundamental change.

Not so long ago in Western society, to be respectable, a woman had to marry as a virgin. This is still the case in some religions. In the 1970s, the sexual liberation movement extensively contributed to abolishing this way of thinking. But when we consider how inhibited young girls remain today when contemplating embarking on their sexual life, we realize the ancestral taboos, which in my day weighed so heavily on sexuality, are far from having been lifted.

"Despite my anxieties," said Marie-Pierre, who had just turned nineteen, "I decided to discover sexuality with a partner of my choice. At first it all went fine, but when we reached the stage of penetration, I froze up completely. Much as I wanted to go ahead, I couldn't, I was closed up, impenetrable. I said to myself that to be free to make love with him the way I wanted, I would have to have my head cut off; I had withdrawn from my desire. He was patient, and we managed to get there. I said to myself, 'Phew! That's done! I'm not a virgin anymore'. I was not sorry, but I was not very happy either."

Regarding this long-anticipated moment, this was how things turned out for Marie-Pierre. Her physical body was surely capable of being penetrated by a man, but her feeling body—that is, her energetic body—went numb and anaesthetized her desire for him. She became obsessed with this blockage. Her feeling body resisted and prevented her desire from gaining the upper hand.

The **vagina**, a supple and elastic canal that ends in a cul-de-sac in the form of a ruff surrounding the cervix, follows. It is made of elastic, pleated fibres, allowing it to adjust to the shape of the penis it is receiving and to dilate in readiness for the foetus to pass through at birth. The rest of the time, it is closed; the edges of the vaginal walls meet. These, like the inside of the mouth, are lined with a mucous membrane, which is covered with lubricating glands. The vagina is where male and female genitals meet, and the pleasure felt there is not just the result of the movement or rubbing together of the vagina and the penis but of an energetic and psychic "intercourse" between both partners' energy and psyche, bringing them into a vibratory rhythm.

The uterus, the fallopian tubes and the ovaries

The **uterus** is a hollow, very powerful muscle made up of two parts, the uterine body and the cervix.

The cervix is a convex cylinder of muscle that opens both ways. In one direction, it lets menstrual blood and babies pass through; in the other, spermatozoa and masculine sexual energy. When ovulation occurs, under the influence of hormones, the cervix opens slightly and secretes abundant cervical mucus, indispensable for carrying spermatozoa into the fallopian tubes and the uterus. Indeed, infertility is sometimes caused by inadequate secretion of cervical mucus or is due to an anti-spermatozoan antibody that cervical mucus sometimes contains. In lovemaking, spontaneously knowing whether or not to allow sexual energy to come through the uterus is, as we have seen, a matter of upbringing and what has been passed on to us; later, it can be learned.

The uterine body is a mobile organ suspended in the pelvic cavity by ligaments allowing it to accommodate pregnancy. It is about 5 or 6 centimetres high, 4 or 5 wide, and weighs about 50 grams. Its capacity goes from about 2 or 3 centilitres normally to 4 or 5 litres in the final stages of pregnancy. Under the influence of hormones, its interior surface is carpeted by a mucous membrane filled with blood, sugar and oxygen, which reappears every month to prepare a nest for a future embryo. If there has been no fertilization it is eliminated in the form of menstrual blood. Bleeding, for a woman, does not mean she is wounded. It bears witness to the fact that she is not pregnant, and that she is a woman.

The **fallopian tubes** are fine, flexible conduits that begin at the uterine horns and end in a fringe-like appendage above the ovaries. The fringes and their mucus secretion take hold of the egg when ovulation occurs. This is where fertilization takes place. Once the sperm penetrates the egg, cellular division is instantaneous. Then, the fertilized egg travels for about three days before arriving at the uterine cavity. The fallopian tubes are the connecting ducts between the ovaries and the uterine cavity; they handle transit. But, as we will see when we consider inherited pathologies, the fallopian tubes are not willing to let just any fertilized egg through. In extra-uterine pregnancy, for instance, fertilization takes place normally, but the fertilized egg fails to migrate; the motion needed to allow it through is jammed. Something is stopping the fallopian tubes from performing their designated task. They are stunned, frozen, they become paralyzed even though fertilization has occurred, the movement necessary to transit from one generation to the next is lacking.

The **ovaries** are our reproductive organs. They produce not just eggs but also the sexual hormones that provide a woman with her "secondary" sexual characteristics: body and pubic hair, breasts, a wide pelvis, the tone of her voice and her sexed appearance in general. Unlike sperm, which is constantly produced and replenished in the testicles, in women a finite supply of ova is present at birth. These eggs undergo many transformations before reaching full maturity. During childhood, some eggs disintegrate without ever maturing; there are 300,000 at birth but only 200,000 at puberty. Then, each month, at the start of a new cycle, which corresponds to the beginning of the menstrual period, about a dozen eggs begin to mature under the influence of hormones, while others decline. Only one egg reaches full maturity (except in the case of non-identical twins). The ovaries are like a bank that keeps a store of eggs, releasing a certain quantity every month, whereas male testicles are more like a factory that produces sperm continually from germ cells.

At menopause, between the age of forty-five and fifty-five, women stop ovulating. Contrary to common belief, a woman's store of eggs has not been completely used up, but her metabolism, which has begun to slow down, no longer allows fertilization: a woman cannot become a mother after a certain age. She still has many eggs, though, which will secrete the minimum amount of oestrogen required for her health as long as she directs the necessary energy to her ovaries.

"I'm lucky: in spite of my many bouts of cancer I still want to make love," Mireille confided. "My vagina has never been dry, in spite of me not taking hormones, which were forbidden." Mireille confirmed that menopause is not, as we are too willing to believe, the end of a woman's sexual life. Yet many women say their sexual desire diminishes at this time of life. This is perhaps because, unconsciously, their desire was fired by the fantasy of becoming pregnant, or by the widely upheld belief that to be a "real woman" sexually speaking is to be a mother.

Hormonal control

The whole life cycle of the sexual system, —maturing of the eggs, ovulation, rhythm and abundance of periods, and procreation, as well as sexual desire—is controlled by the brain. The brain relies not just on hormones but also on neurohormones. The pituitary gland, located in the cranium between the eyes, a spot that Asian medicine refers to as "the third eye," orchestrates the flow of information. It is a matter, on the one hand, of balancing the hormones produced by the interaction between the pituitary gland and the ovaries and, on the other, of regulating the pituitary gland, which is itself under the influence of nerve signals from other parts of the brain, particularly the hypothalamus and the cortex. Hormonal balance depends on all of these organs.

The hypothalamus and the cortex control our perception of self and of the world depending on our history as written into our memory. This is how the state of mind, both conscious and unconscious, influences the secretion of hormones. Malfunctioning hormones are never the root cause of the problems they create but are themselves the consequence of the broader context of one's personal history. Taking hormones to make up for hormonal deficiency allows you to "cure symptoms" for a while by suppressing them but will not solve the problem at its source once and for all. To genuinely re-establish hormonal balance, you have to go through profound psychological and emotional changes that modify how you function so that the brain gives the proper signals to the pituitary gland for it to produce the needed hormones.

The lesser pelvis, the hips and the perineum

"The pelvis creates a belt of bone between the spinal column which it supports and the lower limbs upon which it rests. It is formed partly in the first years of life by the pressure of the weight of the upper body through the vertebrae and partly, as soon as the child begins to walk, by the 'counter-pressure' from the earth on which one stands, through the femur bones of the two legs" (8). The pelvic girdle is formed by the meeting of four bones: in front and on the sides, the two hipbones; at the back, the sacrum and the coccyx, which protect the "sacred space." These bones are connected to each other by four joints, three of which are known as symphyses, i.e., fibrous joints permitting little mobility of the bones: the pubic symphyses and the sacroiliac joint.

The area where the spinal column and the sacrum are joined is especially fragile. This area establishes humans' upright posture. Common complaints like lumbago, sciatica and herniated discs develop from sudden, intense pressure in this area that sometimes occurs when standing up suddenly or carrying too heavy a load without adopting the proper posture. Instead of the body's weight being distributed all over including in the legs, its full weight is blocked at the pelvis, thereby crushing the intervertebral disc. When this happens, you are literally cut in two: with no support from your legs it is painfully difficult or impossible to hold yourself up or to walk.

The pelvis is divided into two parts; the greater pelvis, where the opening of the iliac wings gives shape to the hips, and the lesser pelvis, containing the reproductive system.

The lesser pelvis, a cavity of bone, is closed off at the bottom by the perineum, known to the Chinese as "the muscle of the ancestors" because of its powerful role in the transmission of life, as already discussed. The complex muscular and fibrous anatomy of this muscle creates a horizontal seal that goes from the sacrum to the pubis, resting against the sides of the hipbones. It is composed of many layers, like a double hammock, attached transversally from one thigh to the other and longitudinally from the pubis to the coccyx.

Although its back part is completely sealed, the perineum allows the rectum, the vagina and the urethra to pass through along its mid-line. Its fibrous central core is between the vagina and the anus, at the intersection of all the perineal muscles. Wedge-shaped, the perineum supports the back part of the vagina and is the site of the first *chakra* in Indian medicine. It is layered with transverse, longitudinal and diagonal muscle fibres, which become circular at the anal and urethral sphincters. These layers are the shape of a figure of eight, with an upper loop that encloses the clitoris and a lower loop that encloses the anus. This is why anal contractions are felt in the clitoris and conversely clitoral erection causes the anus to tighten.

The pelvic floor, another term for the perineum, provides the ground support for our organs, without which they would literally fall out through our lower orifices. Besides keeping our organs inside us, this floor supports us by transmitting the earth's dynamic forces from below to above, which give us the strength to carry ourselves upright.

The perineum is an elastic, flexible muscle, allowing the openings it protects to be sometimes firm in order to contract and sometimes supple in order to become elastic and dilate. The perineum plays an important role in our sexual life because we use it to make love—to let the genitals meet and interpenetrate. It is also the muscle which the foetus must confront and push through to enter the outside world.

The Chinese call the perineum "the muscle of the ancestors" because the memory of our origins is concentrated in the perineum. It is not only where our paternal and maternal lineage is rooted but also the repository of all our archetypal, ancestral memories. The imprint of our unique origins is, in effect, inscribed in each one of us.

By stimulating the perineum, we imprint it with new memories, the new memory of our identity, so that it acquires muscle tone, suppleness and elasticity. This can be achieved by contraction exercises, but principally by awareness. Paying attention to the perineum allows us to feel it, "imprinting" new sensations and leaving within us new memory traces called "engrams."

While there are now methods of electrical stimulation to rehabilitate the perineum, the results are sometimes disappointing. This is due to lack of instructions about active participation so as to become aware of the sensations. Of course, this imprinting also occurs through having a sexual life. If you are too preoccupied by problems in experiencing pleasure, fear of not experiencing any or shame if you do feel it, then you withdraw into yourself instead of allowing yourself to be open to the memory that resides in the perineum. This is how the locks of family and societal upbringing remain closed, leaving you oblivious to the body's memory of pleasure and blocking access to the inner, secret garden which is meant to come with adulthood.

Breasts and breastfeeding

In Western medicine, women's breasts are considered "secondary sexual characteristics." This shows to what extent Western medicine ignores the dynamic and erotic aspects of the body. Like all the body's orifices, the breasts have a double function: material and vibrational. Their material function is to produce milk to feed offspring, in their capacity as maternal glands. But the breasts are also communicating organs that send and receive energy. Fondling the breasts resonates in the genitals. In this respect, breasts have a feminine, energetic and sensual function. Firm and rounded, erect nipples attract and invite the "game of clouds and rain," one of the terms in ancient China for sexual intercourse.

During breastfeeding, the sensations of mother and child come into resonance. This resonance will later permit the child to "engram" welcoming and receptivity for the purposes of her future genital sexuality.

Changes and transformations in a woman's body

A singular aspect of a woman's sexual life, from puberty to menopause, is its cyclical nature, mainly expressed through changes and transformations in her body. The rhythm of the lunar cycle governs her time of fertility. Her menstrual period appears approximately every twenty-eight days. Every month, her sexual organs bleed, both because she is a woman and because she is not pregnant.

In most traditional societies, this loss of blood is seen as a process of cleansing and purification, and therefore, during this period, a woman must take special care of herself. However, the bleeding should not be too abundant; it should not cause too much fatigue, since its function is to remove the materials accumulated over the month from her body. If she bleeds too much, she will lose too much energy and enter an abnormal process, as discussed below on the topic of inherited pathology.

It is not normal to experience pain in the abdomen, or to bleed heavily: this causes anaemia. It takes three weeks for red blood cells to be replenished by the body. If a woman bleeds excessively, her body will be constantly overworked renewing its mass and volume of blood during the latter part of her cycle, between the twenty-first and twenty-fifth day. The body always gives priority to life-sustaining functions. Blood is our life fluid. So, it is no surprise that women who bleed too much during their period are constantly exhausted.

When a woman is pregnant, her uterus becomes the womb in which a new being is constructed. It changes shape to make room for this being. Becoming a mother is a major transformation affecting the entire body. The uterus is not where the child comes from but rather a place where he or she is accommodated. The child's origin is the fruit of a spermatozoon fertilizing an ovule, but it is also the fruit of the parents' two life histories, including all the mystery underlying their coming together.

Many traditional societies believe that this coming together involves not just the spirit of the two parents but also that of the child-to-be. Françoise Dolto speaks of a "third desire," that of the child, which, as part of the desire of each of the two parents, is necessary for the child to be born. In this sense, the child chooses the family in which s/he desires to come into the world.

Setting sexual energy in motion

Sexual energy can be called forth in two different ways: either through actual, person-to-person communication with the partner of one's choice, or by means of a fantasy requiring a personal scenario.

When the genitals engage in real communication, person to person, they experience the pleasure of exchange by actualising each partner's sexual energy. Through this dynamic process, we increasingly come to know both oneself and one's partner. We are present both with self and other.

In contrast, during sexual fantasies, arousal is stirred via images. These images, created during childhood about sexuality when no one told us any better, have become the only representations of sex we may have. Through such images and scenarios, our sexual arousal "switches on" bringing pleasure. Yet, when personal fantasies are used to climax, sexuality cannot evolve because it relies on these fixed images and scenarios from the past and hence is repetitive by nature. In these fantasies, we relate only to ourselves. We both want and need a partner, not to be in communication with him, but in order to act out our personal scenarios.

For a fulfilling, dynamic sexual life, you must first be confident, peaceful and happy. Then you can welcome your partner's sexual energy within you and focus on the sensations of pleasure that come with penetration. We will see that this state of mind depends on sex education which, unfortunately, most women have not received.

A woman is not altogether feminine, and a man is not altogether masculine. Each possesses a degree of both feminine and masculine energy, making each of us a unique personality with unique achievements.

A man loves a woman because he finds in her what his own physical body prevents him from developing in himself. Making love is not just for the purpose of getting inside a woman's body so he can assuage his needs and express his own energy. It is also in order to draw on a woman's energy to revitalize himself. The Chinese say that Yin, the feminine principle, nourishes Yang, the masculine principle, while Yang energizes Yin, iteratively on and on. In Chinese, "Yin Yang" means "making love." We can see how Chinese civilization considers the complementarity of men and women. For a woman, the energizing process of sex is not limited to welcoming and receiving masculine energy. She also has the power to mentally project herself into a man's body to join his energy with hers and strengthen the intensity of their coming together.

Sex is not a gymnastic performance. Above all, it is a form of energetic and psychic communication. The best part of love is when you let go. That means allowing yourself to be overwhelmed, so that something new can happen to you. You need to accept the unknown and let yourself be inhabited by something that is not part of you: the life force of your partner's genitals. It is the meeting between his life force and the life force of your own genitals that opens the door to this incredible pleasure that overwhelms you. Making love is not a constantly repeated act that is separate from the rest of life. It is a process that unfolds, gets better and expands with age and experience. It refines one's knowledge of self and other.

Notes

1. Cystitis: inflammation of the urethra and of the bladder, producing a constant need to urinate.
2. See Didier Dumas, "L'origine des troubles sexuels du monde occidental," idem, *Et si nous n'avions toujours rien compris à la sexualité?* (Paris: Albin Michel, 2004)

3. Chia Mantak, *Le Tao de l'amour retrouvé. L'énergie sexuelle feminine*. Paris, Guy Trédaniel, 1990. Translated as *Healing Love through the Tao—Cultivating Female Sexual Energy* (Rochester, VT: Destiny Books, 2005); Jolan Chang, *Le Tao de l'art d'aimer*. Paris, Calmann-Lévy, 1977. Translated as *The Tao of Love and Sex: the ancient Chinese way to ecstasy* (Penguin Books, 1977); Catherine Despeux, *Immortelles de la Chine ancienne* (Paris, Pardès, 1997).

4. This is what the immortal Su Nu told the Yellow Emperor when asked if one could do without sexuality since it is so complicated.

5. Catherine Despeux, *Taoisme et corps humain*. Paris, Guy Trédaniel, 1994. Translated as *Taoism and Self Knowledge* (Leiden: Brill, 2018).

6. See Françoise Dolto, *Sexualité féminine. La libido génitale et son destin féminin* (Paris, Gallimard, 1996).

7. "Co-penetrate" or "compenetrate" is a translation of the ideogram TONG, which expresses the meeting between the feminine breath and the masculine breath.

8. R. Merger, J. Levy and J. Melchior, *Précis d'obstétrique*, 6th edition. (Paris, Masson, 2001).

CHAPTER THREE

The barrier of fire: recurrent disorders

Acute ailments, recurrent ailments

"My genitals hurt so much!" Nathalie told me, beside herself. "They itch and burn! It's awful. I feel like tearing them out. My doctor prescribed some medicine, but each time I think I've got rid of the problem, it starts again. It's really getting to me, especially since I have a new boy-friend. I don't know—maybe I should have further tests to find something that will cure me once and for all."

I have been hearing this request ever since I began my gyn-aecological practice. Every day a gynaecologist is confronted with irritated sexual organs, abdominal pain and bleeding. Nathalie's problem was a version of what had been troubling Catherine seen from another angle.

"Just because medicines cure does not mean they offer a per-manent solution, Nathalie. This is not to say that the medicines are ineffective. As you pointed out, they soon make you feel better. But medicines cannot prevent a problem from return-ing. They can cure you once you are ill, but they cannot reach the root cause that makes the illness come back. You cannot expect them to do something beyond their power," I replied.

Like any medical practice, Western medicine has its limits. Over time, this medicine has become specialized in high-performance, cutting-edge technology, and remarkable ongoing advances in research. Western medicine can identify what is wrong in most cases, which is very important because knowing what has happened to us helps us to take better care of ourselves. Western medicine offers effective surgical and pharmaceutical treatments that focus on illnesses and their symptoms.

However, if a disorder is recurrent, the patient can no longer be treated impersonally, her history disregarded, because a recurrent disorder is always an expression particular to that individual. Indeed, that is why it keeps coming back.

"Your thrush infection, Nathalie, cannot be not treated with different medicines depending on whether it has appeared for the first time or is recurrent. Although, the treatment can certainly be changed, since several equivalent medications are available, that will not really address the problem. As for conducting more thorough examinations, in your case they might be useful to confirm what any experienced practitioner would have already diagnosed. I am not saying further examinations should be avoided, since they can attest to a tangible reality, which is reassuring for both the patient and the doctor. But to treat the yeast infection as something with an external cause, for which more effective drugs can be prescribed so as to prevent a "relapse," is a waste of time. For that, you need a new frame of reference, because Western medicine is not competent in this area.

"There are, and always will be, all kinds of parasites both on us and in us. As long as they are cocooned as spores, fungi do not cause trouble. The fungi troubling you, Nathalie, are like those growing in nature. They can grow and develop if they find themselves in a warm, damp place. It is certainly important to know how to treat them, but you also need to know how to avoid providing them with a fertile breeding ground where they can proliferate."

It took me many years to realize I had to look at a disease differently when it was acute versus when it had become recurrent and chronic.

Looking for the origin

"Let's put your endlessly recurring thrush problem aside for a moment," I suggested to Nathalie, "and talk about you. When did this problem appear?"

"It developed gradually. Just after the holidays, I think. At first, it wasn't too bad."

"Was it before or after you met your new boyfriend?"

"Come to think of it, it was right at that time. The first time Jean-Marc invited me to dinner at a restaurant, just the two of us. I even said to myself, 'Well, this is a great start! Then I forgot about it. He and I had known each other for a while at the university, but we had always gone out with friends."

"You seem to like him."

"Very much. We have so many things in common. We love to do things together. Really, this thrush is a drag!"

"And when did you have thrush for the very first time in your life?"

"Oh, that was something! I was on vacation at my grandmother's house. I was thirteen years old. I'd just got my period and was with a group of friends who met up every year. I didn't dare say a word about it to anyone, until I couldn't stand it anymore and had to ask my grandmother for help."

"And the first time you got your period, at thirteen. How was it?"

"I hardly had any cramps. I wasn't surprised, since my mother had already explained what would happen. She told me that she didn't want to be like her own mother, who'd told her nothing, so that her period had come as a shock. She hadn't dared to speak to anyone about it but had promised herself then that she would be sure to warn her own daughter once she had one. So, she simply told me that I would have my period, that I would bleed once a month, that it was normal, that I shouldn't get upset, and that nowadays there are all manner of things to protect yourself!"

"And your sexual life, when did that begin?"

"I was pretty young when I began hanging around with boys, but I really wanted to choose my first boyfriend carefully. I chose someone I really liked, we agreed to have sex—and I was disappointed! It's true we weren't too experienced, but even with time it never got much better."

"What exactly disappointed you?"

"I don't know what I was expecting. I imagined all kinds of amazing feelings that I had never felt before."

"Did you have an idea of how sex was for your parents?"

"No idea. It was never discussed in our house. Do you think that has something to do with my problem? My mother is a fairly withdrawn person, not too demonstrative. Anyway, I found out recently that she wasn't too 'keen on that sort of thing', as they used to say back then. Sex was something you had to resign yourself to. She believed that some women were "keen on it," while others, like her, were not. Basically, it didn't bother her. She didn't need sex."

"And your father?"

"Not a word about anything like that ever came out of his mouth. He was very quiet, too. All I know about my father is his work."

"And your grandparents? Do you have any idea about how sex was for your grandmothers?"

"I never even thought about that! I have no idea! My grandmothers were both pretty straitlaced. My mother's mother was great with me when I was very little. She was a domineering woman, and for as long as my grandfather lived, she was the one who wore the trousers. If there was a love scene on television, she inevitably made fun of it and commented on how disgusting it was. My mother's father was very self-effacing, but very nice. He spent his time tinkering in his workshop, where I loved to be with him. As for my father's mother, she was widowed very young, soon after her marriage, when my father was still a little boy. She was sober, strict, immaculately tidy and always in mourning. So far as I know, she never had anything to do with another man."

"The place where the body expresses itself by experiencing pain is symbolically significant. A stomach-ache is a sign that something in life is "hard to stomach." Constipation shows you are keeping something inside which is no longer doing you any good and which needs to be eliminated. Trouble breathing means something is stifling you. Leg pains indicate trouble going forward in your life. Migraines come from incoherent thoughts that clash with each other and clutter the mind. For you, Nathalie, the problem is sex.

"Your thrush first appeared when you were thirteen, just after your first period, at the moment when sexual energy begins to express itself in the body. You were on holiday with friends, staying with your grandmother. Your body was expressing the impossibility of you enjoying your sexuality; you are coming up against that same grandmother's ban on sexual pleasure. This is the taboo that made your mother frigid and, in your case, has caused recurrent thrush. You do not need to be with your family for this problem to manifest, because it is already inscribed within you. You want to make love with your boyfriend and feel it is legitimate because you are living in a permissive society. but what you don't realize is that the women in your family continue to prevent you from doing so."

Fire in the genitals: blocked sexuality

"Your genitals are on fire, Nathalie. The fire of sexual desire is obviously present. But instead of being a nourishing fire that lends you wings to set about lovemaking with the man of your choice, a taboo turned the fire into a destructive one, setting up a barrier of fire between you and Jean-Marc which has made you unapproachable and unable to delight in the coming together of your bodies.

"Your life force is clearly strong. It allows you to open your heart to Jean-Marc. It allows you to discover each other and to expand your shared life. Your sexual desire could open your genitals to invite your partner inside you, filling you up with life force with the discovery of yourself and your partner. But instead, your sexual energy turns against you, as if your grandmother's disgust toward sexuality was stopping you from enjoying your own.

"Thrush reveals how you have remained prisoner of your little girl status, unable to move on to becoming a woman, because nobody ever explained to you that one day you would come to live your own sexuality."

"But why should I be forbidden to have sex? I want to make love with Jean-Marc!"

"Your desire and your heart, Nathalie, might have wanted to make love, but the cells of your genitals did not. It was as if those cells, which contained your grandmothers' memories, were stopping you. When children see love scenes on TV, it makes them wonder what is happening. At that moment, it is important that adults not be evasive. It would seem that the mockery and disgust of your grandmother regarding sexuality made you choke back your questions and that as a result you later behaved as if you had no genitals.

"The information about sexuality that was inscribed in your cells when you, as a little girl, were being constructed was coming from your mother "sex, haven't the faintest"; coming from your maternal grandmother, it was "sex is unpleasant and disgusting" while from your paternal grandmother the inscription was "sex is nothing, it's a hole, it's empty." All these messages ran contrary to your desire for Jean-Marc, with the result that

34

your genitals got itchy and began to burn, like they did the first time at your grandmother's house. Since your mother renounced sexual pleasure, you are the first woman in the family to try to enjoy life as a sexually fulfilled woman.

"Meeting Jean-Marc, which meant a lot to you, reawakened the memory of this basic sexual construction that shaped you, so powerful and unyielding that it still controls you. Without realizing it, you remained true to that memory."

Loyalty to one's mother is a very strong link affecting a woman's sexual construction. This is partly because our mother made us, and partly because our body resembles hers so that, in order to become adult, we spend our childhood identifying with her.

"The taboo against sex," I explained to Nathalie, "does not come from your own thinking. It is the result of the way sexuality was written into you and unconsciously handed down."

We inherit these messages. They are imprinted within us and form our basic structure, which is made up not only of our own thoughts and beliefs but also of our "cellular memories."

For centuries, female sexuality has been yoked to reproduction, while the pleasures of the flesh were vilified. Things were still this way when I was young. In terms of sex education for children, nothing has fundamentally changed. Sexuality is still not handed down from mother to daughter as a human value, indispensable to human life and health. The result is that women like Nathalie, who want to experience their sexuality, do not succeed. Because their mothers never said a word about erotic pleasure, their cells are not prepared for it.

"So, there must be tons of women like me," commented Nathalie.

"Tons!" I agreed. "The right to integrate sexual pleasure into everyday life is a recent social phenomenon, a change that has come with the contraceptive pill—even though the pill was invented to keep the birth rate down, not so that people could make love as they choose. Your mother could have taken the pill herself and discovered her own sexuality, but she never felt entitled to do so. As she told you, she never felt the need for sex. Desire never even reached her genitals. It was not part of her body. Her upbringing had completely extinguished desire. Your ailment, thrush, is a way of protesting against this disastrous legacy. Take it as a sign of progress.

"The capacity to feel the desire to make love depends on what is handed down, starting very early in infancy, by the men and women in our family whom we love and most especially by our mothers. Your upbringing could not teach your cells that sexual pleasure is normal. Like your mother and your grandmothers, you are still governed by past memories. Your life is still not determined by your own choices.

"As with most recurrent disorders, your thrush raises a series of questions: 'What's all this about irritation of the genitals? Why do I always have thrush? Why do I develop thrush when I feel desire for a man?' It signifies something that you did not know—'I didn't realize my genitals don't really belong to me but are still anchored to those of my maternal ancestors.' Not only a medical disorder, it is also an invitation to break this pattern—'I didn't know I had all this work to do in order to feel happy as a woman.'"

It took me a long time to understand that when an ailment resists all types of medicine and keeps on coming back, we have to revise our conception of the ailment and of the treatment. The disorder shouldn't be seen as an enemy to be battled against, but as a teacher telling us to reclaim control of our life.

Chinese medicine

Let us consider Nathalie's thrush from a different medical viewpoint: traditional Chinese energetics, acupuncture. Chinese medicine holds that life comes from forces called "vital breath" (*Qi*), that enable us to move, nourish us, bring us to life.

36

When these nourishing and protective breaths are able to circulate harmoniously in us as they should, we are healthy. If there are too many or too few of them, we fall ill. At death, these breaths leave our physical body. We become cold and motionless. Life has left us.

In Nathalie's case, the conflict created by the fact of being in love and the fact that her body lacked information needed to make love caused humidity and heat to build up in her genitals. The energy of sexual desire did not know which way to go. It had no direction, so it went around and around in one place and ended up seeping out of her body. Sexual desire produces both "hot blood" and "moist genitals," therefore providing fertile ground for a flare-up of fungus. Sexual energy began stirring restlessly on the spot, itching and creating a barrier of fire that pushed her partner away and turned against Nathalie herself chafing her terribly.

Chinese medicine treats this condition by getting the energy to circulate, dispelling the humidity, and cooling down the heat. This allows the breaths to move freely again. For immediately treating acute symptoms, Western allopathic medicine, homoeopathy and acupuncture are equally effective in the short term; it is up to each individual to choose the one that suits best. But if, after being cured, the disorder recurs, we need to do some personal therapy work to acquire a new state of mind that will prevent the slightest emotional upset from bringing it on again.

Disrupting the repetition

Nathalie had to learn to separate herself from the process which caused her disorder to recur; she had to enable herself to live by her beliefs and feelings, to let her desire carry her beyond what had been handed down to her about sexuality but was no longer what she wanted for herself. She had to realize that sexual fulfilment was made taboo by her family, and that the thrush expressed the absence of a sexual construction that would let her live out her desire. She would also have to educate herself, allowing new imprints that legitimized her sexuality.

To achieve that, I propose to my patients overall energy work which calls on imagery, inviting them to feel the base of their abdomen like a basin that needs to be full of energy. This is our base, our reservoir of life energy. Within this basin are various organs. It is beneficial to mentally contact and feel them: the kidneys, the adrenal glands, the ovaries, the uterus, the vagina and the perineum. Then, feel the energy in this reservoir overflowing in abundance, going over the thighs all the way down to the feet. Once in contact with the perineum with our feet on the ground, we are steady, upright, and no longer adrift. With this stability, we can connect—mentally—to the forces inside the earth, the forces that make plants grow, so as to bring these breaths back up into the pelvis. These forces support us, carry us and straighten us up. They reshape us so that we become more completely ourselves.

This transformation cannot be forced wilfully onto one's life. In the long run not only would that not be effective, it would be dangerous. Instead, it is a matter of "intention," of "wanting" it firmly, and of staying focussed, remembering one's eventual goal. What brings about transformation is the desire for transformation. It is the intention and attention we bring to them that make these exercises work. Nathalie's desire to become a vibrant woman enabled her genitals to become reintegrated into the rest of her body, allowed her to become supple, open, and welcoming, so that the barrier of fire was extinguished.

Making love

What is especially senseless about the way we approach lovemaking is how deeply we have internalized the thinking handed down to us. I was fourteen when a girlfriend first said to me, "Making love is really amazing!" I couldn't get over it! I had never heard a woman talk that way about the sexual act, and I never thought you could dare try it unless you were officially committed to a man. I was speechless but instead of seizing the opportunity to find out more, I was shocked and dumbfounded. I thought that at seventeen she was too young! In short, I simply blanked out what she told me back then. It was not until later, thanks to my own therapy sessions, that I understood why I could not accept my first lesson in sex education. It was unthinkable that a girlfriend should be the one to inform me of the existence of such pleasure because at that point in time, I was unable to call into question what I had learned at home. My mother, who wanted to bring me happiness, and always told me that I was "a beautiful girl," couldn't possibly have overlooked such important information—if it were true, she would have told me so! How could I have imagined that she herself had never explored herself as a woman?

Looking back, I can still see myself sitting on the front steps next to my girlfriend and hearing her say "Making love is really amazing!" I looked at her. I felt a tiny stirring inside myself that threw me off balance, and I could no longer hear what she went on to tell me. Still I hear the ever-receding echo of those words, pushing back the boundaries of my world: "Making love is really amazing!" There was me, entering into a new world. But all of a sudden, a black screen obscures my face, preventing me from seeing this new landscape. I hear my friend again but from a great distance. When I gather my senses, a moralizing speech forms in my mind. What was it that happened then, without my knowing it? Françoise Dolto would say I fled to my "secure base." Fleeing to that place, which provides the comfort of the "known," is a spontaneous defensive reaction which occurs when you are incapable of taking in something so new that it emotionally overloads you. The black screen was saying to me, "Don't go any farther. You won't be able to handle it."

At that age, to be able to really hear what my friend was telling me, the idea of sexual pleasure should have already existed in my family and been available for sharing between my mother, my sisters and me.

Teaching our genitals about pleasure

So long as a woman's genitals have not been informed of their pleasure-giving function, they do not know how to come to life. The ability to produce offspring does not teach you to make love. But that's what happens. Being true to one's original construction and in particular to one's mother is an extremely powerful bond for a girl.

In her own mind, sexuality was not taboo for Nathalie; she did not consciously believe she should not make love with her boyfriend. The taboo came from the attitude towards sexuality handed down and inscribed in her. We are all imprinted by what was handed down to us to create our basic structure, and this is the origin of our "cellular memory" and of what we think and believe.

Until my generation, which saw the advent of contraception, people were told that life consisted of working and having children. It is still like that: sexuality in itself is still not presented as something of value to humanity. Nathalie thought it would be good to make love with the man she loved, but the cells of her genitals were not inscribed with this idea; they remained sealed off in her "original matrix."

Until the 1980s, psychoanalysis was the only tool I had found to expand my ability to treat others and to treat myself. I could not ignore the mind's influence on health and behaviour, so I soon tried to find reasons in my patients' lives and past history to explain their illnesses. Disorders are warning signals, telling us something we are unaware of but need to know. So, I looked for a specific event, recent or from the past, that had upset my patient to the point of undermining her health and making her vulnerable. Was it bad news, a change in circumstances, a marriage, a family visit, meeting someone new, moving to a different place, some bad luck, a death, a birthday, a birth?

I adopted the contemporary psychoanalytic thinking of Françoise Dolto, who has studied preverbal development in very young children, taking into account their heritage and re-establishing that a baby is a desiring being in his or her own right from the moment of conception. Parents, or whoever is responsible for children, have not just the right but the duty to tell them the truth about their history, what is unique to them, as well as the history of their family and ancestors. All of this rightfully belongs to a child. It is at the root of their psychological and emotional health.

Parents must tell their children what the parenting plan behind their birth was, how they themselves were conceived, what it was like in the family during the pregnancy, as well as the circumstances of their birth and the first years of their life, of which they have no memories of their own.

All these facts, feelings, sensations, thoughts, beliefs and values, as well as the individual or collective achievements of her family, constitute the "original matrix." From this matrix a child draws the materials that make up their mental structure in the form of engrams (1), the cellular imprints of the child's perceptive and emotional life. This initial structuring of physical, emotional and mental character builds the basic feeling of safety which, on becoming an adult, fashions sexual behaviour.

Adult sexuality, eroticism and the emotional rapport with a partner are constructed in the first years of life, using both the information contained in the "original matrix" and the words used to inform them. It's therefore primarily through "mothering," which transforms thoughts, emotions and sensations—whether the person mothering is the mother, father, big brother, sister, grandparents, or nanny—that we hand down the way they will handle sexuality later on. Secondarily but simultaneously, "fathering" converts thoughts, feelings and sensations into words that can be said by all the child's carers.

The life force that inhabits us

In the West, we say "My life lies ahead of me." The Chinese say, "Life inhabits us." To this way of thinking, thrush, like all recurrent female complaints, signals that the genitals are not inhabited by life and are unaware of how to achieve that state. Acupuncture gave me a representation of how the breaths of life, which I also call "energy" or "vital forces," animate the body and circulate through it. Acupuncture has helped me to know myself and to dare consider the role of sexual fulfilment in health. Yet, it took me quite a while to get a clear idea of the different forms of pleasure that are produced in the clitoris, the vagina, the uterus and the rest of the body.

Thrush, vulvitis, vaginitis, cystitis, salpingitis, oophoritis and pyelonephritis all come from an excess of fire, which manifests in inflammations of the genitalia and the urinary apparatus. All these disorders are evidence of dysfunction in a woman's body that stems from a lack of sex education. In terms of energy, these inflammations bear witness to how women have been raised without being told about sex. As little girls, they could not imagine themselves as women who would have a life of sexual pleasure. Their life choices indicate their desire to fulfil themselves, but when it comes to freely experiencing their sexuality and sharing it with a partner, their body tells them that in certain ways it remains stuck in the past, and that this past wins out over their desire.

Most mothers and fathers no longer repress the sexuality of their children. But they still neglect sex education because they lack the words to talk about desire and sexual pleasure. They enable their children to grow up, to choose an occupation, and to start a family, but they have not properly equipped them to become sexual adults, responsible for their emotional and sexual lives.

Note

1. This term, which I have already cited in an earlier chapter, is used by Françoise Dolto to describe the way in which emotional events are imprinted in cellular memory. According to the theory of origination developed by Pierre Aulagnier and Didier Dumas, the foetus and the young infant construct themselves as both self and other simultaneously. In this way they duplicate their mother's mental structures and also those of her loved ones, in order to emulate the aims of the other [i.e. her mother's loved ones], a process which forms engrams. When a person is described as a "sponge" regarding her external environment, she is going back to this original structuring, which enables her to empathize when someone else is suffering.

How little girls construct their sexuality and how daughters come undone when their mothers die

Expecting a little girl

One beautiful spring morning, Veronique came to see me. She was feverish and exhausted, with inflamed sinuses. She announced that she was four and a half months pregnant.

She told me there were no problems; everything was going well—she was happy to be expecting a child and to share her life with her partner.

I pointed out that, considering the state she was in, something had obviously upset her.

She blushed and said, "Last week I had an ultrasound exam and found out I'm going to have a girl … It's great! Greg is so happy!"

"And you?"

"To be honest, I would have preferred a boy."

Veronique was very emotional, on the verge of tears. I was well-acquainted with her personal history, so I said to her: "Your older brother is already a father whereas your older sister has no children. Your father is doing better than your mother. So, it must be stirring and more complicated for you to have a daughter and become meshed with the women in your family." Ultrasound technology, discovered and put into use only about thirty years ago, makes it possible to know the sex of a child while still in the womb. This is a real revolution. Not everyone chooses it, but ultrasound does enable us to accurately personify the unborn child. We used to speak of "the baby" or "the child": a sexless angel. After an ultrasound exam, a woman is no longer expecting an angel but a little boy or a little girl. Expecting a baby has become gendered.

And what kind of shock operates on the future mother who finds out she is expecting a girl? Well, it is in the expectation of "sameness" and not difference. The extent to which we feel comfortable expecting a little girl depends on how comfortable our own mother felt when she was expecting us, as well as any other children, especially girls. When a woman is pregnant, she reconnects with her mother's pregnancies. She simultaneously relives her mother's state of being pregnant and her own state of being a "female baby." Veronique's sinusitis attests that due to her family history, expecting a girl was upsetting and made her ill.

What might happen within the couple, what solution can be offered today to this couple so they can await their baby girl calmly and happily, without repeating the mistakes of their forebears?

For a couple to experience the best possible pregnancy and birth, they need to know that together they are producing their own particular creation, that the two of them are bringing their child into the world. How they await their child, both separately and together, directs and moulds the kind of parents they will become to this particular child.

I advised Veronique and her partner Greg to take an active part in creating their daughter's birth by practising a technique that is particularly appropriate during pregnancy: haptonomy.

Haptonomy comes from the Greek *hapsis*, which means touch—the sensation of contact—but also sensibility, sensitivity and feeling. In France, haptonomy was introduced in the 1980s by GREEN (the French acronym for Neonatology

Research and Study Group) (1) founded by Dr. Frans Veldman of the Netherlands. They organized the first conferences for obstetricians and pregnant women.

By practising haptonomy throughout pregnancy, right from the *in-utero* stage, the future parents learn to give their child a place of his or her own. If the future mother is willing, by putting his hands on her stomach the father can directly establish contact with his child *in utero*. And the child in turn can respond to their father. An exchange based on "affective touching" is established between father and child.

Essentially, this method fosters the active participation of the father in his partner's pregnancy. The woman is no longer alone with her child. With the father's presence, the three-way dynamic relieves the woman of the powerful connections of the "mother–daughter pair."

But most important is that the parents-to-be share what is going on between them. Fathers now straightaway fulfil their complementary role to the mother. With or without haptonomy, fathers quickly establish contact with their child, and that is what counts. They imprint memories directly in and with their child. As a result, the woman they love is relieved of the all-pervasive maternal function.

At birth, the child becomes the magnetic catalyst

At birth, a child becomes the centre of the world for a mother, a magnet. The incestuous energy bond that a mother feels with her child disconnects her sexual desire for the man she loves: the same love bond is now transferred from her man to the baby. The bonds of the heart and spirit with her beloved, the man whom she has made into a father, are still present, but her sexual love has moved towards her own umbilical centre to nourish her child emotionally. Her pelvis and genitals are no longer vibrant: they are deserted and have ceased to be invested by her. The man, whose sexual desire is still

47

alive, finds his woman sexually lost to him. His virility is no longer cherished.

By resuming their sexual life, parents protect the infant from this exclusive bond with the mother. When that balance is restored, the mother will be regenerated, the father will stand erect, and the child will be able to engram sexuality for the future.

Learning to be a man or a woman at the same time as a young parent is a new situation that our ancestors did not experience. Desire is reawakened when a couple rediscovers the intention and the confidence to sexually celebrate having met each other and the pleasure of having produced a child. Putting aside their maternal and paternal function momentarily, making time to share a moment of intimacy, will restore their joyous appreciation of themselves and of each other. It will radically change the atmosphere of their household.

The power of names and surnames

A child's first name gives him or her a family identity and a social identity. Every day, the baby hears the sound of this name, this particular vibration, when the child's parents talk to and take care of them. This name, which is constantly used to attract the infant's attention, is what eventually leads that child to say "I." Telling a little girl the story behind her first name is useful. Whether the choice reflects a happy memory her parents have shared, an actress they idolize, a tyrannical ancestor or one of the father's former mistresses, the imaginary that led to the choice of the name is of primary importance to the child herself. If it is a name like Morgan, Alex and Chris, which does not mark the difference between male and female, the child needs to know if the parents expected her to be a boy instead, or if the name refers to an ancestor, or if sexual difference was not important in the family.

A little girl also needs to know whether her mother or father in particular chose her first name and if the name refers to some specific event or idea. If she has a name like Sylvie which in French sounds like 'si elle vit', meaning 'if she lives', or Renée which sounds like 're-née' meaning 're-born', does that mean that she was unconsciously conceived to replace another child who died? Transgenerational psychoanalysis teaches us that some first names are given in memory of a child who died before the present child, whether a sibling or further back in the family history.

The surname establishes the child's filiation. In our culture, bearing the father's name is the only proof a mother can offer her child to attest that the child was conceived with someone from a different lineage to the mother's own. Better yet, nowadays it is possible to use the name of both father and mother, documenting that the child issues from both lineages. But if a little girl is told nothing about the origin of her filiation and if she bears only her mother's last name, she could forge her identity in the belief that she was conceived by her mother alone and is therefore only an extension of her mother. This would force her to remain embedded in her mother, believing there was no need for a man to reproduce life.

> Here is what Monique had to say: "Not being legally recognized by my father and not having his name handicapped me for a long time. I completely lacked confidence in my ability to be successful socially and in my encounters with men. As soon as I began a love affair or found a job that suited me, it all fell apart! Then, thanks to therapy, I realized that the reason I was unable to gain recognition socially or from a man was because I hadn't been acknowledged by my father."

Corinne, another of my patients, never brought her pregnancies to term. Genealogical research enabled her to discover and understand how her ancestors had borne children. Her great-grandmothers and her maternal grandmother were all their "mothers' daughters," and, from mother to daughter, they fitted together one inside another like Russian dolls. From generation to generation, by giving their own name to their daughters, they showed that, unconsciously, they believed their daughters were conceived by parthenogenesis and that a man was not needed to conceive a child. Corinne's work with energy and transgenerational analysis enabled her to accept that the child she would give birth to would bear the name of the father Corinne had chosen.

To fully realize you are a woman, you must also see it reflected in a man's gaze and first of all in your father's. If a girl has no father, her relationship with men is bound to be problematic.

Breast-feeding

Genital awareness is also assimilated through breastfeeding: the nipple is the first object of penetration through the mouth into the body of a nursing baby. The nipple is the representation, the hinge between the baby's outer body, bounded by the skin, and the inner body with its functioning organs.

Suckling allows babies to discover their body's internal autonomy because, inside their mother's womb, even though they were already sucking their thumb and swallowing amniotic fluid, they had no sense of the difference between inside and outside. They merged with that aquatic environment (2). Suckling triggers inner sensations by combining satisfaction gained from filling oneself through the mouth and the enjoyment of this liquid as a continuum with the mother's pleasure in nursing her child.

For a mother, breastfeeding brings about uterine contractions (which used to be called "after-pains" because they are sometimes very painful). These contractions help the uterus regain its prior tonicity and shape. Giving birth and breastfeeding, which give rise to the contractions, bring about a transformation in the woman's perception of her uterus and vagina. If the transformation is experienced as positive, pleasurable and well-received, she will then enjoy a more mature and fulfilling sexuality.

The exchange that takes place during breastfeeding constructs a secure base for the baby. Her mother's smell, the brightness and depth of her gaze, the physical closeness that gives support and comfort, not to mention her mother's reassuring and restorative voice: with all of this, the little girl is completely nurtured.

For these internal sensations to prefigure future utero-vaginal climax for the baby girl, her mother must both acknowledge them to herself and communicate her pleasure to her daughter. That way, her daughter will let herself feel these same sensations in sexual climax with a man later on. The mother should also express to her daughter, using words, that she herself and her foremothers could not allow themselves to freely feel these sensations, because it was not permissible in their time.

During nursing, if a mother suffers from cracked nipples, lymphangitis, breast abscesses, swelling or a lack of milk, the baby's first penetration by the nipple will be fraught with difficulty. These pathologies show to what extent, involuntarily, the new mother is affected by the maternal problems of her female lineage. For her baby daughter, these two mouths, the oral and the vaginal, resonating with each other, will no longer have the confidence to welcome and receive nourishment from her mother. Later it will make it hard for her to enjoy kissing or welcoming a man's penis into her body. The vulva, the vagina and the uterus are cut off from their source, the oral mouth. The genitals are no longer irrigated and become dry and insensitive, as if anaesthetized.

When the uterus of a newly nursing mother remains oversized and lacks tone, her spirit is, unconsciously, still pregnant. It fails to give her uterus the signal to resume its cycle. Lacking the information to be sensitive to erotic pleasure, the breast can only take pleasure in feeding. Such a mother remains "psychologically pregnant," failing to re-emerge as a new sensual, sexual woman.

If there are problems breastfeeding, if the baby girl gets either too much or not enough milk, later when she is a young woman, she may reject the penis—or, on the other hand, never be able to get enough of it. She will take it in as if to fill herself, but she will not truly desire it.

There was a time when breastfeeding was frowned upon because it risked spoiling the beauty of a mother's breasts. A wet nurse was preferred as if breasts were totally interchangeable. This is a complete denial of the intimate and privileged relationship between the child and the breastfeeding mother.

Nowadays a baby's bottle may substitute for the mother's breast. The bottle can play the same role as the breast if the mother verbally explains to her new-born why she is using a bottle: "I don't know or understand why I can't nurse you with my breasts, but when I know I will tell you. Meanwhile, let's share the pleasure of your feeding: enjoy your milk." Words spoken truthfully will always release a child from her mother's problems.

Today, fathers also give the bottle to their child. This way, they share the feeding role with the mother. For the baby, this establishes the maternal function both through the mother and the father, which is fundamentally structuring for the baby because affective encoding derives from both parents. It is important to note, though, that some doting fathers are so infatuated with their baby that they abandon their gendered role as men. They risk becoming "emasculated," in a similar manner to the risk of "defeminisation" for women. In both cases, sexual desire disappears.

Building the baby girl's sexuality

A mother does much more than give birth. She literally fashions her daughter's future. She makes it possible—or impossible—for her daughter to be sensitive, secure, educated to become a happy woman and happy mother, capable of exercising both these functions. Like all human abilities, sexuality is contingent on receiving the knowledge and know-how handed down to us. The construction of femininity is handed down by women. It is their job to teach their daughters what it means to be a woman.

The goal in instructing a daughter is to plant the seeds of her future femininity, to allow her to embed in the cells of her body the dual role of her sexuality: that of pleasure and sexual fulfilment, which will make her feel like a woman, and that of reproduction, which will induce her to become a mother. The information on which her sexual construction depends will be modified and evolve as she grows up. Most important is to bear in mind that a girl needs to be aware that she is destined to become an adult.

In our culture, it is tacitly understood that a mother knows how to hand down to her daughter the pleasure of becoming a mother. This is far from the case, as is demonstrated by the existence, in France, of a "motherhood training department," directed by Dr Jean-Marie Delassus, where mothers who have not been handed down that knowledge are taught to be mothers. In contrast, what fails to be considered is that, for a girl to later be happy as a woman, femininity too must be handed down.

For a little girl, the curtain of the theatre of life opens out on to her predestination to become a mother but also a woman "proud of the genius of her genitals." Women of my generation did not know that being a mother and being a woman were not the same thing.

Becoming a mother does not automatically imply becoming a woman. Different energies are called on and different objectives are sought: the feminine function and the maternal function are not performed in the same space and time. A woman is not the same person when taking care of children as when making love with the man she loves.

Freud theorized the sexual construction of boys. Unfortunately, his theory was also applied to girls. Until Françoise Dolto remedied the situation (3), therapists saw the sexual construction of girls as one of helplessness and loss due to lack of a penis, as if they had no genitals of their own. However, if a little girl is informed of what her body is like, i.e., like her mother—her woman's anatomy will not be degrading for her. On the contrary, she will understand that she is different from her father, her brothers and men in general, that she is complementary to them, and that the genitals of a man and the genitals of a woman are made to fit together like Lego bricks. Just as a little boy needs to know that the function of his testicles is to give life, and that this function travels through his erect penis, a little girl needs to know about her clitoris, her vagina, her uterus and her ovaries. In fact, if she is free to express herself, she will say: "I have an hole and a button" (4).

Our society still fails to integrate that adult sexuality is constructed out of the body-to-body affective experience of the first three years of life. A little girl builds herself, just as a little boy does, from what her parents are, how they consider her and take care of her. Her parents are the models she uses to construct herself. Their family history, their way of life, their state of mind, their thoughts and beliefs will teach her and allow her to develop. The way they look at her, speak to her, touch her, wash her, feed her, change her, talk to her or answer her calls is what structures and shapes her physical, emotional and moral growth. It constructs her "sense of self" (5) and her "secure base."

Through all these exchanges her body will take in and be imprinted with the knowledge of her various future functions and capacities. All this affective language will consolidate as her memory. These exchanges literally mould a girl, following successive phases of construction and integration that enable her to become herself.

Before she can talk, her first information comes to her as an undifferentiated mass. A little girl cannot yet distinguish the exact meaning, but she can tell the difference between pleasure and displeasure, interest and disinterest, kindness and unpleasantness, coherence and incoherence.

The dyad stage

In her first three years, a little girl develops within the psychological space of her carers. She has not yet separated from her parents. This period is called the "dyad" phase. For the psychoanalyst Didier Dumas, this is the phase of "origination" (6), when a child duplicates not just the parents' language but also their mental functioning and sometimes their "transgenerational phantoms." The little girl constructs herself within the geographical and interpsychic space of the people who take care of her. She does so by picking "information blocks" from the pile that her environment offers and integrating them into her actions. She assimilates the customs, ways of thinking and emotional and sexual structures of the adults with whom she identifies. This is how she comes to mentally resemble her parents.

Sorting the information occurs through a classification system which, at this age, is binary. For a baby and a small child, things and events are either "good," or "not good," pleasant or unpleasant. So, the little girl selects whatever she finds to be most suitable and most empowering, in order to incorporate that information into the structure that makes up her personality.

In this way a baby girl constructs her first representation of herself, of her personality, and of her genitals. She finds confirmation of her intuited femininity, on the one hand from her parents' pleasure or displeasure at her being a girl and, on the other hand, through the sensations she feels in her genitals.

These sensations of pleasure come from physical and emotional exchanges with her mother, her father and her other guardians when they take care of her body, especially the erogenous zones of her mouth and genitals.

With her mouth, it is the way they feed her, talk to her, babble and sing with her, and let her discover the world by putting things in her mouth. With her genitals, it is the way they wash and bathe her: a little girl discovers her sex when it is touched, washed, dried and cared for. Female mammals always clean the genitals of their young by licking. Humans care for the sexual organ by bathing, drying, lifting and generally helping the child to feel comfortable.

These attentions create specific sensations from which a baby girl constructs erotic feelings. They will procure different feelings if care is given with gentleness, respect, calm and consideration as compared to mechanically administered gestures. And the sensations that come from bodily care leave their mark on a little girl just as much when her mother or father washes her as if her genitals did not exist—by not touching or even thinking about them—as when they are coveted. Such nonverbal messages are imprinted in the cells of a baby girl, creating "engrams." Ignoring or, on the contrary, paying too much attention to her genitals interferes with the construction of her body image and "sensorial skin."

It is the fact that her genitals are recognized as what they are that enables a little girl to regard them as a natural part of herself.

In this environment, she learns to walk, to speak, to put together sentences and to think. She is taking the first steps in becoming humanized. She is aware of existing, she is able to open herself to the world, and, at about two-and-a-half, she gains control of her sphincters. Everything is in place for her to grow up and become an "unfrigid woman": she can talk, she no longer needs nappies, she can move and be autonomous and has the confidence of a little girl already prepared to experience the pleasures of her future life as a woman. But she has not yet acquired the capacity in her body for welcoming and receptivity.

A little girl first expresses her emotions and feelings according to the system of values of her nearest and dearest. During the dyadic phase, a mother who takes pleasure in making love and in being a mother automatically transmits these feelings to her daughter. But it is not often that a mother prides herself on the genius of her genitals or those of her partner!

Nowadays, parents no longer explicitly forbid their children's sexuality. Nonetheless, since most of them have not been constructed in this manner themselves, this natural transmission celebrating sexuality cannot be accomplished properly. Being the perfect parent is not the point. It is a matter of being sincere, of knowing how to talk about yourself and your own childhood. If information is missing from what has been handed down, the parents can bring it into existence simply by talking about it, thus immediately dissipating that lack of ancestral transmission. Words fill in the gaps suffered by the parents. With words, parents mark their daughter's energetic foundation with what she may need to properly construct her future sexuality. A mother can say to her daughter: "I will teach you to be happy to be a girl, even though I myself didn't know that I could be happy to be a girl, and I still haven't managed to do so."

Telling one's children the truth about one's feelings saves them a lot of time by helping them to know where they stand in their own lives.

Wanting to know the true story

At about age three, when children enter a new phase of life which psychoanalysis calls the Oedipal phase, they need to know how they were conceived. The little girl wonders about the desire her parents felt before her conception. This is the age when she discovers that she came out of her father's testicles and her mother's ovaries. She wants to understand her father's role in her arrival in the world, especially if he is not there, or has separated from her mother, or died.

If she was adopted, the little girl needs to know why and to hear about her birth mother (7) and her birth father, even if she learns that she will never meet them. It is certainly very important to know that her adoptive parents welcomed her with joy, but the most fundamental point, upon which her future health depends, is to know the truth about her past.

If she was born after a brother or a sister who died, or even after a miscarriage, it is important to tell her so. This informs her of her position amongst her siblings; for her parents too it is important because by talking about it they will differentiate her from the child who died, and help her avoid confusing herself with the one who was unable to live. This will prevent her from becoming a "replacement child," with ensuing psychological risks (8).

She also needs to know what her mother's pregnancy was like, with its anxieties, if any, or the family problems that arose during the pregnancy. Parents' ailments that appear during pregnancy have to do with stumbling blocks in their own family history, which confront them when they contemplate their future parenthood. The labour and birthing processes should also be described: if the child had the umbilical cord around her neck, if forceps had to be used, if her mother had to undergo a caesarean. If as a newborn she was ill, kept in an incubator or hospitalized, the little girl needs to know how she was treated there, what the family atmosphere was like around her cradle, who she looked like and what people said about her.

Of course, the little girl should not be emotionally invaded or flooded with useless information, but it is important to be aware that she has been affected by the circumstances and feelings surrounding her arrival in the world. The correct words will enable her to match the symbolic realm of feelings with actual feelings she perceives. This coherent relationship between what is said and what is felt will allow her to construct a unified self. As an adult, this congruence will allow her to experience her body and be able to express herself while making love.

It is a mistake to spare her from the hard truths of life so as to avoid hurting her. On the contrary, the absence of words will close her off in her own mental world, unable to connect with what she feels. Only the truth will allow her to acquire what she lacks. If the truth is hidden from her, when she grows up, she will feel lost without knowing why, torn between her thoughts and her feelings, as if she were always waiting for the mysterious information that her parents never gave her.

Finding self-recognition

Hearing her parents talk about her, a little girl perceives her value and feels that she exists. If her parents tell her she is wonderful for doing so many new things, that she does them so well and therefore she is surely growing up, she will feel confirmed in her activities. With them, she learns to know her body and to name all its parts, including her genitals. So it is important to explain to her that her vulva and her clitoris are just the external parts, that the vagina, the uterus and the ovaries are inside, and that when she grows up she will be able to experience the pleasure of being a woman in her tummy and have children.

It is ridiculous, though quite usual, for parents to explain sexuality in an abstract or scientific way that steers clear of the topic of pleasure. Such explanations leave out the sensations a child experiences in her body and the questions those sensations raise for her. If a mother sees her little daughter touching her genitals and enjoying it, the mother needs to say, "That's the place that really makes you a girl. You are like Mummy. You will enjoy being a woman" (9). If no word is said about the pleasure that comes from her genitals, erotic touching can become compulsive, without the little girl having any idea of what is happening to her. Talking about masturbation as something natural, on the other hand, confirms her status as a girl and allows her mother to acknowledge her daughter's future status as a woman. A simple but relevant word is enough to reassure the little girl and stop her from losing contact with the outside world by fixating on the excitement of touching her genitals.

As she grows up, her mouth and her genitals become substitutes for her relationship with her mother. Thanks to her mother, these parts of her body were the first sites of enjoyable exchange. If her mother explains how she is built and gives her permission to explore further on her own, the little girl will be able to also explore other aspects of life. She will not be compulsively attached to her genitals. Except when it helps them sleep, children masturbate only if they are anxious or bored. In addition to words, the goal of a little girl's sexual education should be to help her discover the mobility and agility of her whole body, something that later will allow her to feel comfortable as a woman.

The father's role and the difference between sexes

During early childhood, children integrate their gender by identifying with the parent of the same gender: a little girl constructs herself by identifying with her mother while a little boy identifies with his father. In identifying with her mother, a little girl projects herself into her own future as a woman. But since at this age her universe contains only her parents, she makes sense of the desire for her father by wanting him to give her a child. "When I grow up," she says, "I'll live with Daddy and we'll have a baby that I'll push around in a pram." In this way she learns to anticipate the future, even before she has fully grasped the idea of time. By imagining that she can be her father's wife, the little girl becomes a person differentiated from her mother.

Hence, she leaves the dyad that together they had formed until now. There is no point in explaining to her that what she imagines can't be done. Instead, it is necessary to reassure her that she is growing up. Her mother, too, was once a little girl who, like her, wanted the same thing with "Grandpa," her own father. That did not prevent her from meeting another man.

At this age, the father's role is no longer to care for his daughter as he has done up until now, but to allow her to understand that he and her mother do not have the same life forces and they therefore do not have the same function. He is someone other than her mother. The fact that she was created means her two parents are different: his life energy is in his testicles; her mother's is in her ovaries. These two forms of energy meet in the mother's body, showing that the father's energy is outgoing, travelling from the inside of his body towards the outside, while the mother's energy is receptive, arriving from the outside and moving inside.

After her mother, a father is his daughter's first object of desire. His presence protects her and helps her stand erect as she constructs her future desire for a man. He is the other half by means of which the girl exists. For a child, there is no such thing as a father without a mother or a mother without a father. Each makes the other possible; each creates the other. One must never lose sight of this: in daily life, the roles of the mother and the father are always interwoven and only exist by virtue of each other, whether or not they live together.

A father is as important in the construction of a girl as he is in the construction of a boy, because it is through the father that the daughter differentiates herself from her mother. A woman who has not been legally acknowledged by her father or who has never been able to live with him has a hard time finding her way in life. She may remain locked in oneness with her mother,

61

as if her mother created the daughter just for herself. Or else, she never finds a man or is incapable of living with one.

Through their father, children discover the outside world. A father is proof that life consists of more than a mother. He opens the doors of the world to his child. He gives his child the "tools" which will enable the child to know how to manage on their own. In this sense he separates the child from the mother.

The fact that a man does not carry a child within his body allows him to carry the child in his mind. His relationship with his daughter is brought into being therefore more through the mind than the body, such that she uses his ideals, values, thoughts, and desires to shape her own. Yet, to construct herself properly, it is important for her to have physical closeness with her father while she is a baby. A little girl who was carried, changed and cuddled by her father will not be afraid of men when she grows up. If she was taken on her father's lap and held in his arms, she will not be afraid to snuggle up against a man. Entertaining a tender relationship with her father as a baby will give her "cellular knowledge" of masculine energy. When she falls in love with a man, she will reproduce this energy exchange, discovered as a young girl with her father. All the more so, if she was able to find the keys to femininity with her mother.

What makes a man a father is his pleasure and pride in having a daughter. How he sees her as a future woman and a future mother necessarily determines her sexual life, because the way he sees her shapes how she matures into a woman. However, so that the daughter does not remain fixated on her father, she needs to renounce the idea of becoming "his wife." A father must be aware of this and express it. This is what is called "the age of reason" or "the end of the Oedipal phase." It is important that a father lets his daughter know that he is glad she exists and that she will be a beautiful woman when she grows up, but it is her mother whom he wants as a wife.

It is through her mother's eyes that a little girl discovers how important her father's genitals are for her mother. And it is through her father's eyes that she sees her mother as a woman (10). Her father must, therefore, speak to his daughter of his love for her by saying "I will never love you as I love my wife, because you are my daughter" (11).

The incest taboo is a universal law which, in order to preserve the succession of generations, forbids sexual relations within a family. It concerns both parents, because when there is incest in a family the mother is always complicit, whether or not she knows it. In those situations, we always find unacknowledged incest in both the paternal and maternal lines. Incest denies the notion of generations causing severe trauma. Explaining the incest taboo to a little girl at an early age, rather than avoiding it, will protect her from being crushed between her generation and the previous one, later enabling her to meet men without shame or guilt. She will then be able to appreciate a man's company and feel like a woman, not a sexual object.

Just as it is important for a mother to let her daughter know that sexuality is regenerative and that it is a pleasure to be a woman, it is important for her father to do the same: he should come forward as a man able to attest the benefits of sexuality. Regrettably, women often discover their father's sexual life only when he dies. "Finding out about my father's hidden sexuality," one of my patients told me recently, "allowed me to discover sexuality myself." Men, too, often remain stuck in the sexual examples set by their father and grandfather, that is a sexual desire split between "the mother and the whore." If a father's sexuality is split, he either experiences it as unspeakable or decides that his children do not need to know about that side of life. He will not find it easy to explain to his children how sexuality has benefited him in his life. Men like this are often painfully silent. Sometimes they insist on applying stringent rules utterly unsuitable for raising children properly and put across a forbidding impression. Some are violent, irritable and angry, or impossibly remote and rigid, as if they do not know how to be alive, loving, generous and glad to have children.

These unbending attitudes often signal there is something to hide. When they are older my patients discover that a father had mistresses, a double life, other children they had never heard about, hidden male lovers or that their father was a celibate priest and so could not live with his children. My patients also sometimes discover that a father was silent because he no longer enjoyed any sex life at all. Perhaps the arrival of children and the repetition of transgenerational patterns drove him into a "vacuum," or perhaps his own father's absence left him completely depressed, whether or not he realized it.

The heaviest burden that a father may place on his daughter's sexuality, whether he means to or not, is to disallow her encounter with other men: he wants to keep her all to himself and therefore slyly presents himself to her as a sexless being. Either he fears the power of women, or he projects onto his daughter his own feminine element, which he was unable to enact, or never dared to do so. In other words, unable to accept his own femininity, he wants his daughter to do so for him.

Telling a little girl that later her genitals will welcome a man's

When her daughter is between the ages of three and six, her mother should tell her about the pleasure of growing up, not just of becoming a mother but also a woman. The little girl cannot know that pleasure now since she is still too young, and cannot experience it by herself, with her mother, father, or anyone else.

From the age of three, with the acquisition of speech, a little girl can begin to separate her own psychological space from that of her parents. So, it is important at that age to give her a representation of life and of sexuality that will enable her to establish a coherent connection between what she feels and speech. In this way, she will be able to put words to feelings. Being able to talk about them with her mother is what enables her to feel unified and coherent in herself.

Without these words, the expression of sensations is repressed. As an adult, she will have a split sexuality: she will know how to give and to enjoy caresses, but her sensitivity will all remain on the surface of her skin—as soft as a baby who cannot be penetrated. In the arms of the man she loves, she will enjoy the pleasure of reunion with her baby skin, unaware that she can and must open herself to receive the energy of his genitals inside her.

Reliving those gentle, delightful caresses are no longer what she needs; it is, rather, something new: the unknown that enters and passes through a woman when her genitals and those of a man meet and fit into each other. A little girl needs to understand that an adult pleasure awaits her, when she grows up and is attracted to someone who reciprocates. This is a pleasure that enriches our life and makes it more interesting.

At this stage, a mental process occurs that embeds the difference between men and women, their complementary roles and functions. Knowing the difference and integrating it teaches the girl about life's realities. This is what enables her to separate her energies from that of her parents when she reaches adolescence, propelling her towards life, towards new encounters, and towards her existence as a woman, as well as enabling her to survive the death of her mother.

Parental intimacy

A little girl needs to understand how each of her parents is strengthened by the intimacy they share, and she needs to discover this over the course of time through what her parents show her. This way she will understand that sexuality is not just about reproduction but also about pleasure. If her mother says, "Your lover's penis will get big and strong when he is inside you, and you will be very happy, as I am now with your father," the little girl will certainly want to experience it for herself later on.

Children are always thrilled when adults kiss in front of them, showing their closeness, their joy in having met. So many of my patients complain of the cold, asexual atmosphere surrounding them in childhood, how their parents never made the slightest gesture of tenderness or sensuality towards each other! Parental functions are asexual, and most parents stay within those limits. All they allow their children to see is the image of a mother and a father who continue to think, like at the start of the twentieth century, that it is improper to talk about sex in front of their children as if that would traumatize them. Whereas, in fact, the parents' role is to explain life to their children.

Excluding sexuality from the family atmosphere is a mistake. Without being exhibitionistic or immodest, parents need to show that sexuality is part of life. In this area, a father has a role to play in making sure he and his wife have room for intimacy. For instance, he might say to his daughter "Find something to do for a while, because your mother and I want to be together to make love."

Even if a mother lives alone or does not have a fulfilling sexual life, she should let her daughter know: she might say, "I didn't know it would be hard for me to have a sexual relationship with men, and with your father in particular. I've learned things since, and I hope you will learn how to enjoy your own sexuality."

When parents have a life-giving sexual relationship, the family atmosphere is different. Contentment reigns in the household, and everyone is part of it. This affects the future too: a little girl is being loved for what she is. She is not repressed if she talks about sex. She is free to be curious about the world, and with time she will feel more and more empowered.

"But where was I before?"

In answer to this question, if parents tell their little daughter that before her birth, they were already thinking about her and wanting her, she will light up. When they raise their child, parents must answer not only questions about sex but also questions about death. If a little girl understands that she can exist in someone's thoughts, words and desires, she can see that there are many ways of existing. This way she can accept death, telling herself that after death it is possible, as it was before birth, to be connected to those you love even if you no longer see them.

Past generations have constructed a taboo against talking to children about death. Lifting this taboo lets us realize that we are mortals and allows our children to realize it too. Children should be permitted to attend funerals. Taking part in a rite of departure allows them to understand that their parents are the extension of their grandparents, and that they themselves will be the extension of their own parents. In this way they can incorporate the transgenerational dimension of life into their thinking.

A little girl knows what she is doing when, seeing her mother's jewellery, she delicately asks, "Will that be mine one day?" We need to know how to answer this kind of question (without feeling insulted at being hurried into the grave). We can tell our daughters, "I don't know if all my jewellery will still be here. I may have given some of it away. And you might have to share some if, by then, you have a brother or a sister. But you will certainly get some of it." By answering her like this, she can imagine herself as an adult.

This is above all the age of asking questions and of "whys." It is the age when a little girl constructs her own values. So, it is disconcerting for her if she does not get an answer. We could say that we do not know, that we never thought about it before, that we will try to find out, or that she can ask someone more qualified. No one is expected to know everything, but we must neither pretend to know what we don't nor evade her questions. A child must never be left in the lurch.

If two adults whom she cares about—her uncles, her aunts, her friends or her parents—disagree, it is a good thing, provided they do not quarrel about it, because it allows a little girl to think for herself. Pretending not to have heard in order to elude her questions, as adults often do, is untenable because parental incoherence is passed on to the little girl who in turn becomes incoherent herself.

The questioning phase is temporary. It usually does not last beyond the age of six or seven, by which time a little girl should have accepted that she will not live with her mother or her father all her life. From then on, she can contemplate having fiancés, sweethearts or favourites, without feeling guilty and without pitting this love against her love for her parents. Her parents must discreetly consent to this new love.

When a little girl reaches the age of reason, at seven, she enters what Freud calls the latency period, a time when she is not concerned with sex. All her curiosity goes into her relationship with girlfriends and towards social, cultural, artistic or sports activities. Sexuality is no longer the centre of her life.

The arrival of her period once more places her within her female lineage. She needs a good understanding with her mother to achieve this transition easily, to be enthroned and propelled into the world of women. To give her daughter confidence, her mother will need to adapt her own language and behaviour as her daughter develops. The mothers of my generation were not socially prepared to act naturally or to talk about such things with their daughters, not having themselves received those benefits from their own mothers or from society.

The age of thirteen or fourteen is when permanent teeth are in place. In this new body, where a young girl does not yet really feel at ease, she discovers a smile in the mirror that helps her to see herself as a future woman.

The bottomless pit: falling into depression

"When my mother died, I lost my connection with the man I loved. Just before she died, when I realized she was dying, I stopped being his woman, without really noticing it was happening. I was sucked into a deep pit. I was no longer myself. I wasn't there anymore," Armelle told me.

No matter how old she is, a woman often falls apart when her mother dies. Her mother, the model on whom her own construction was based and to whom she remains attached, has disappeared. She is not prepared for this loss. The maternal connection is still so powerful that a mother's death causes her daughter to lose her foundation and her energy structure. Even if she is already an adult and a mother, indeed even if she is a grandmother, she collapses. It is truly earth-shattering. Her usual landmarks disappear. Unmoored, she finds herself catapulted into a no-man's-land. She becomes someone else: lost, fragile, tiny, defenceless.

"I didn't want to get dressed anymore," Patricia said. "I stayed in my dressing gown. I didn't leave the house. I had nosebleeds, headaches, constant nausea. I was incredibly weak. I could no longer move. I was sick every morning and I could only eat if I was given anti-nausea injections. I was obsessed with how everything alive decomposes: I watched rotting fruit and vegetables. I deliberately let cockroaches invade my house. Day after day, I scrutinized how the mould spread. I myself was in the process of decomposing, but I didn't realize that until later. I didn't even say to myself, 'I am crying because I've lost my mother'. I said to myself, 'I'm nothing'. I had no life left in me. I no longer wanted to make love. I didn't want to be desired as a woman. I was no longer glad to be a woman. I wanted nothing at all."

A mother's death is an unexpected blow that plunges you into a bottomless pit, causing you to lose your "secure base," your landmarks. You are no longer a woman. Either you are no longer there, or you have become nothing.

Such a collapse calls into question the way your entire adult life has been constructed. You believed yourself to be free, independent, living the life you had chosen, but suddenly your mother disappears, and you no longer exist. That is when you realize how the invisible tie to your mother has remained surreptitiously powerful: you continue to be an "occupied territory." Your mother was "your everything," and her death leaves you incapable of any other loving connection.

The intensity of the depression that a mother's death brings about—because it really is depression—depends on the personal energy foundation a woman constructed until then: how she has constructed in herself the woman who works, the maternal woman who raises children, the woman who is desired and who feels desire, her relationships with her family and her friends, and her relationship to spirituality.

If a girl is not introduced to the idea of death before she finds herself in mourning, whole sections of her personality will no longer function as before. Certain parts will become lifeless and be invaded by "phantoms," taken hostage by the unmourned spirits of previous generations.

Patricia was to realize later, during therapy, that her collapse was the result of two bereavements that were never mourned: her own loss as well as the bereavement suffered by her late mother who was only eighteen months old when she lost her own mother and had therefore never properly mourned her.

Another of my patients, Marie-Claude, also collapsed when her mother died. She came to understand that her situation was similar:

> "My mother never mourned her own mother, and neither did my father. I already knew that, and thanks to

my analysis I integrated that knowledge. But when my mother died, the way it hit me took me by surprise. I no longer took the slightest pleasure in life, I was completely adrift, and I went back to my analyst to get my moorings. My sorrow was my own, but my collapse came from elsewhere. I had fallen into the abyss that had swallowed my mother up when her own mother died, a hole from which she never climbed out. I was swamped by the mourning that never took place for my mother's mother, my maternal grandmother, whom I had never known."

The way a girl falls apart when she loses her mother is all the more severe when she inherits unmourned loss(es) of her grandmother(s). She becomes submerged by the enigmas of her past.

Marie-Claude became aware of her feelings by means of a dream: "I was in a dark, vertical tunnel that had no floor. I floated in this vertical tube. I went up and down without knowing where I was. I saw my body, made of a thick, light-grey mist. I was fascinated. I wanted to know where I was. I couldn't get out. I had been huddling inside myself for months, losing all my strength. I hadn't been aware of time passing. Then I realized that I had been enclosed in a space where I was emptying myself of all my energy."

It took Patricia much longer to get out of her deep depression: "I couldn't talk to anyone about my pain. My husband said, 'I don't know why you're letting yourself get into such a state. Your mother was ill for two years. You knew she was going to die!' My best friend said, 'You did everything you could! You knew it was coming. You knew she was on her way out'. Yes, I knew it, but I hadn't experienced it as a reality. I didn't know I would react so violently and lose myself to that extent. In the end, I wasn't prepared. I felt nobody understood me. Friends who had not lost their mothers were dumbfounded and didn't know how to help me. I was like a robot on automatic pilot. I didn't even feel my own pain. My personality had vanished."

Quest for meaning and renewal

Then Marie-Claude happened to read a man's description of his depression after losing his wife: he said you must not linger too long in such a state "because that is how you get ill." Marie-Claude told me, "I knew what he said was true. I became aware that I was dying, probably to reunite with my mother. Suddenly, it became obvious. It was unbelievable: I had lain in the arms of death without realizing it! After that, I had to decide whether or not I wanted to live. It wasn't so much that I decided to live, but I decided not to sink into illness, not to become a burden to my family and my friends. That was how I got back a little of my own taste for life. Not getting ill became my driving principle. If I remained in this debilitating fog, I would never recover. I had to change my thinking and my behaviour, find the strength to get out of that abyss that darkens everything. I began writing down what was happening to me. I started to feel better, but the desire to get well was not enough. I needed more strength to pull me up and to rediscover my roots in living reality. I realized I needed help to find this extra strength."

As for Patricia, she had decided to die. She was waiting for death when the wish to leave something for posterity rallied her. "No, I couldn't die right away. First, I had to write about why I want to die. I discovered the pleasure of putting words on paper. This pleasure made me realize that I didn't want to die, and it also showed me strengths in myself I didn't know I had. I was filled with an extraordinary energy that pieced me together again. Since writing had brought me to life, I held onto writing, and it became my pillar of strength. I had never written a screenplay in my life. I began to write one, something I'd always dreamed of doing. I sent it to a competition, and I won. I became a screenwriter and a filmmaker. That's why I could say many years later that by departing early, my mother left me a real gift. Her death showed me who I was, whereas before, even if I thought I was doing what I enjoyed and found interesting, I was still enacting part of her desires, living for her."

A mother has an immense responsibility towards her daughter. She not only shapes her daughter's future, but she must propel her daughter out into the world and away from herself, give her the wherewithal to become independent. If a mother fails to show her daughter how to be independent of her mother so as to be able to construct herself as an adult woman, her daughter will remain under her mother's sway and, when the mother dies, her daughter will collapse.

For her daughter's sexual construction to be as it should, a mother must work on her own sexuality. And for her daughter to construct an independent life as an adult woman, it helps for her mother to look into her own transgenerational past, to build her energy foundation and to discover her own true history.

Mothers and daughters are an extension of each other. They contain each other, there is no severance. Our ability to procreate means that the bonds of love transcend death. It really is a case of Russian dolls: I contain my mother who contains her mother who contains her mother, and so forth. Our mother gives us life and calls to us when she dies. We have been her "everything" and she has become our "everything." Life without our mother is meaningless. If we continue to contain her, she dies within us.

To put an end to this endless spiral, we can state today that before contemplating giving life, a woman should create an energetic and transgenerational foundation strong enough for her not to need to interfere in her daughter's life. The more stable a future mother's foundation, the less she will keep her daughter under her sway.

Women who are grandmothers today have had contraception available and, over the course of time, have taken on board the different stages of women's liberation. They have a role to play in handing down family history, thereby strengthening the energetic foundation of their granddaughters, passing to them what they were unable to give their own daughters.

Notes

1. GREEN: Groupe de Réflexion et d'Évaluation de l'Environnement des Nouveau-nés.
2. See Jean-Marie Delassus, *Le Génie du foetus. Vie prénatale et origine de l'homme* (Paris: Dunod, 2001).
3. See Françoise Dolto, *Sexualité feminine, op. cit.*
4. Dolto, *Sexualité feminine, op. cit.*, p. 157.
5. Françoise Dolto, *Le Sentiment de soi, op. cit.*
6. See Didier Dumas, *Et l'enfant créa le père* (Paris: Hachette Literature, 2000); idem, *Et si nous n'avions toujours rien compris à la sexualité?* (Paris: Albin Michel, 2004).
7. Closed adoption, which deprives a child of the right to know who her mother or father was and is, from this point of view, a shameful practice, that continues to apply in only one European country: France.
8. See Anne Ancelin Schützenberger, *Aie, mes aieux! Liens transgénérationnels, secrets de famille, syndrome d'anniversaire, transmission des traumatismes et pratique du génosociogramme*, 17th edition. Paris: Desclée de Brouwer, 2003. Translated as *The Ancestor Syndrome: Transgenerational Psychotherapy and the Hidden Links in Family Tree* (London: Routledge, 1998) and Didier Dumas, *L'Ange et le Fântome. Introduction à la clinique de l'impensé généalogique* (Paris: Minuit, 1985).
9. Françoise Dolto, *Sexualité féminine, op. cit.*, p. 157.
10. Didier Dumas, *Et l'enfant créa le père, op. cit.*
11. Françoise Dolto, *Sexualité féminine, op. cit.*, p. 16.

CHAPTER FIVE

The gynaecological family tree

With inflammations that create a barrier of fire, we saw how our genitals have not received the legacy needed for opening up to a lover. Now we will see how, when our genitals are obstructed, painful, ill, sterile or fertile at the wrong time, they carry disorders inherited from our female lineage. We inherit from those who brought us into the world. With them and through them our genitals take their place in our body and acquire their functions. We inherit their strengths along with their weaknesses.

Painful menstruation

"As a young girl," Josiane told me during an office visit, "when I had my period, all I could do was lie down with a hot water bottle on my stomach. That was the only time my mother took care of me."

"Did your mother also have painful periods?"

"Yes, but her mother told her not to be such a sissy. My maternal grandmother was a stern woman who worked hard. She herself never had pain with her periods. It was her older sister whose periods were painful, and only the heat of a clothes iron relieved her."

"And you are also the eldest, like your mother and like your grandmother's sister. In your family, the eldest girls are the ones who had painful periods, and that pain is handed down from one generation to the next."

When we study "gynaecological family trees," we find repetitive behaviour like this, with women inheriting the same problems as those whose position in the family in past generations was the same as their own. The symptoms and the intensity of discomfort are not necessarily exactly identical from one generation to the next, but their repetition points to the fact that each woman is affected in her own way but that the problem is a family line disorder.

In Josiane's case, the great aunt, the mother, and the daughter suffered from the same problem, but they reacted and responded each in her own way, according to the mores and the means available at the time. The great aunt used a clothes iron; the mother had to ignore her pain; the daughter got relief from a hot water bottle and her mother's affection.

Women's lives can therefore be punctuated by pains that rule their existence in a regular, repetitive way. Many women complain of such problems:

- "In the days preceding my period I'm always depressed, and when my period comes, I feel completely drained."
- "My stomach gets bloated. I feel heavy and weighed down."
- "I want to experience my womanhood calmly, without stomach pains. My period is hell, especially when it comes during the night. In the daytime, if I keep busy or work, it's not too bad, but at night it starts up. It's always the same nightmare. In the days before it arrives, my spirits drop, and my desire plummets to zero."
- "I'm sick of having a tummy ache every month. It brings back the demons that haunt me."

When women tell me about their painful periods, excessive bleeding or premenstrual syndrome, I suggest we make an inventory of the female problems in their lineage. It is not normal for a natural process to be painful. Having a period is not accidental or unexpected. Bleeding does not signify a wound. It is a sign of femininity and of the absence of pregnancy. For a young girl, the arrival of her period for the first time is a transformation, a leap out of the world of childhood propelling her into the discovery and the construction of her future as a woman.

Certain women experience very painful periods or heavy bleeding every month like a storm, a tidal wave, a cyclone or a flood. Something is intruding in their pelvis taking over and overwhelming them. Other women, instead of abdominal pain, have terrible migraines.

These pains hit women, handicapping them for several days each month, claiming much of their energy, making their lives exhausting for them and for those around them. In my generation, the most common explanation mothers gave to their daughters was: "It's normal for it to hurt. It will stop when you have a child." This is far from the truth. At that time, no one was taught anything about the nature of menstrual periods. Few mothers told their daughters they would menstruate one day. This is what happened to Nathalie's mother, who had no idea what was going on and thought she was dying.

Here are some of the things my patients' mothers told them when they first got their periods:

- "It's nothing at all, darling."
- "You're a big girl, you are becoming a woman, and you will always feel bad. It's normal."
- "You'll have to be careful, now. All men are bastards."
- In tears: "My poor little girl."
- "What did I do to have a daughter who's suffering so much?"

- "God, will you ever stop growing up?"
- "So, what did the teacher tell you at school?"
- "Listen, be sure to wash out your towels in the bidet."
- "Now, you are a woman: Watch out!"
- "No more freedom for you. You're not going out anymore."
- "Already! But you're so young …"

After being spoken to like this, how can a girl possibly see the arrival of her period as a positive event marking the start of a new life as a woman?

The luckier ones were congratulated, but I could count them on the fingers of one hand: "We were a family of five. When a girl got her period, she would receive the gift of her choice, which we all went to buy with our parents. I chose a wide belt with a beautiful buckle." In a world where we no longer use rites of passage, this is a fine way of helping a girl to move forward into her adult life.

It is important to warn a young girl that she will begin to menstruate. She needs to know not only what will happen to her physically but also what this new status represents and implies. Physically, she will bleed every month. The blood comes from the uterus and flows through the vagina. There is nothing to be embarrassed or ashamed about. This is the physiological functioning of the female body during a woman's reproductive period when not pregnant. It is not dirty and disgusting "old blood"; it is a mucous membrane engorged with precious blood, the blood which nourishes the life in a fertilized egg prior to the formation of the placenta and which is expelled when fertilization has not occurred.

Of course, a girl should be prepared for this expulsion of blood. Nowadays, there are all manner of "protections" available, a message the media are constantly drumming into us. But what is most important for a young girl is not to deal with the bleeding but to realize she is moving into a new mode of functioning.

When her period comes, a young girl's mother should quietly honour and support her, commemorating the occasion by wishing her daughter a happy life as a woman. The arrival of a young girl's period should be neither hidden nor broadcast to the whole world, but it is the time for a mother to tell her daughter how it was for her and for other women in the family. A mother needs to realize that her daughter has to know about the sexual life of the women who came before her. The arrival of her daughter's period is the opportunity for a mother to talk about her own life as a woman. In fact, if she herself was traumatized by the coming of her period, she may not know how to simply tell her daughter she will grow up and have to leave her mother in order to become a woman. A mother's intention is not to upset her daughter, but if sexuality has not been simple for her, she probably does not know how to talk about it in simple terms. She does not know how to tell her daughter outright that she too is a woman. It does not even occur to a mother who has been unhappy in her life as a woman or a mother to wish her daughter a better life than her own. But that is the only way to help a girl save time by daring to get beyond her mother's problems.

If her mother says nothing, a girl automatically finds herself caught in a net of indefinable inherited stumbling blocks that overwhelm and paralyze her. It is very hard for a girl to do better than her mother unless her mother permits it. But this permission has to be genuine and heartfelt. A mother must speak from her heart, from her feelings, and tell the true story. If her words are true, they will reinforce her daughter's secure base. Like a house that needs strong foundations to support its walls and roof, a daughter's foundation is consolidated by this information. It becomes embedded in her, and she will be able to build her own life as a woman. The information is imprinted in the cells of her body and genitals. Now that she has been made aware of her own history, she is in a position to get on with her life.

Another benefit that comes from a mother speaking in this way is that she will be able to accept that her daughter has grown up and can no longer be "her little girl." Mothers too need to separate from their daughter and detach themselves. It is one thing to be glad to see one's daughter growing up and doing well, which shows that a mother has completed her mission. It is quite another to detach oneself from one's daughter and trust her in the knowledge that she no longer needs help.

Letting her children go is an integral part of being a mother. Hanging on to them holds back their growth. If a mother is unhappy or feels abandoned, to support her mother a daughter will remain attached to her and be unable to live her own life. A mother has to learn not to need her children in order to stay alive. She needs to find other ways to engage with life. Letting go of them is a real transformation. It is not always easy, because the maternal function has been to help, nourish and support her children while the children cannot do these things for themselves. A mother has devoted a whole slice of her life to this necessary role without taking sufficiently into account that it would not last for the rest of her life.

There are also mothers who were unable fully to give themselves over to the maternal role. Having themselves lacked either a role model or the necessary maternal force, they could not support and contain the child's needs. Too agitated or too fragile, these "child mothers" or "absent mothers" have an aversion to the maternal function. They throw themselves frantically into other activities, absenting themselves from their child. They let go of their daughter too soon. The daughter, lost, needs to cope with this lack of support and create ways to survive so that she does not fall apart.

Lacking a secure base because she did not get the kind of attention she needed, a young girl may later lack empathy. She will grow up without a strong sense of her own existence. Young women like that ask a lot of their men, while at the same time neglecting them. They seem to constantly be trying to make up for something missing.

"Phantom" disorders

Today's young women are no longer ashamed of their period—a real improvement over my generation—so how do we explain why so many women still experience painful periods? Medical questioning reveals that many gynaecological disorders are inherited. Either a woman's mother or her aunts had painful periods, or her grandmother and her great-grandmothers were burdened with terrible problems: hysterectomy; prolapse of the uterus and the ovaries; death due to extra-uterine pregnancy, breast or uterine cancer, or at childbirth; stillborn children; repeated miscarriages; the loss of a mother, brothers or sisters at an early age due to an epidemic, or of a father due to war; orphaned; illegitimate; adopted and ignorant of their own biological history.

In our mothers' and grandmothers' time, nothing was said about such things. No one thought this silence would have future consequences. People kept quiet about tragedies they hoped to forget, as if keeping quiet could make painful memories disappear. It was believed that if everyone kept quiet, children and others would be spared pain. But hiding painful memories does not make them go away. The wounds of life and death—and hence of sexuality—remain open in the unconscious and cannot heal.

It is impossible to come to terms with these misfortunes without having a correct representation of them. When trauma cannot be accepted and digested, it is passed on to future generations, creating "phantom disorders." Secrets and unspoken truths become encrusted in the mind and make it impossible to have a clear vision of life. They create a tomb (1) within, where traumas remain alive and have to be expressed one way or another.

Premenstrual syndrome

"Premenstrual syndrome" is the medical term for the hidden forces carried within us, which express themselves in disorders synchronous with our menstrual periods. For some women it might be a bad mood, vulnerability, dissatisfaction, sadness or violence and having a grudge against the whole world; for others it might be apathy, inertia, exhaustion or depression, not to mention painful breasts, a bloated belly, swollen ankles and legs, nausea and vomiting, or terrible migraines.

By answering my questions, my patients discover how their heritage from their female ancestors weighs on them. I ask them to research the important events in the sexual life of their ancestors, to talk with their mother, aunts and grandmothers in order to find out how they experienced their life as a woman and as a mother, paying attention to the dates of births, marriages, separations, illnesses and deaths to see if there is any repetition.

My patients have learned that their own pain bears witness to the past suffering of women in their family, which their uterus is trying to push out. Painful periods are often like contractions. The lower abdomen may be contorted with pain because it has encountered an obstacle, a knot, an uncomfortable blockage that it wants to expel. The same thing is happening when bleeding is too abundant (2), which is another way the body tries to rid itself of something that gets in its way. Yet there is nothing that needs to be physically eliminated: examination shows these women to be normal. The blockages they encounter during their period are not physical. They are located in the energetic, emotional and mental body and attest to psychological trauma that is still an "open wound." The origin of the problems handed down from mother to daughter is hidden not in the physical body but in the psyche and in the emotions. By talking with her mother or with a therapist, her condition starts to make sense and to be resolved.

Young girls need to be told that they are configured like their mothers and like the women in their family. I have often noticed that this information is enough to relieve their pain. Knowing that our problems are not really ours but come from the past can allow us to take back control of our bodies and put them to rights. My youngest patients add humorously, "So these huge breasts and fat thighs aren't mine either!" Therapeutic energy work can help them regain their figure and a normally functioning body.

Painful or over-abundant periods are an early sign of ailments inherited from female forebears, which are later corroborated by the gynaecological illnesses women encounter.

Gynaecological ailments and their origins

Françoise is seeing me because surgery has been recommended for her fibroma. Her uterus has become enlarged and her periods are abundant and tiring. She would like to try an energy treatment rather than have her uterus removed right away. She is forty-three. By questioning her, I discover that her older sister had a hysterectomy at the age of forty-four and that her aunt, her mother's older sister, also had one at forty-four, as did her mother at forty-three.

Françoise is the second daughter of three children. She is three years younger than her older sister and her brother is two years younger than her. In her mother's generation, there were also two daughters three years apart. Her mother was the second and was followed, after two years, by a haemorrhaging miscarriage. Continuing her work with me, Françoise learned that two generations back her grandmother died in labour at forty-three, giving birth to a boy who did not survive.

Her father, Bernard, was the tenth of twelve children. He was given the same name as the ninth child, who died before he was born, and was followed by an eleventh child, who also died young. Placed between two deceased brothers, Françoise's father had carried death within him since birth.

This information and the obvious repetitions that come out were a revelation. Françoise knew she was following the same path as her mother and sister, but she had not made the connection with the death during childbirth of her maternal grandmother at her present age that no one had told her about. She knew her grandmother had died while her mother was still young, but the circumstances of her death were always avoided. Françoise didn't know that her grandmother died giving birth to a boy who also died. She could never talk about it with her mother, because at the slightest question her mother would sink into deep sorrow and weep. The subject had to remain unspoken. This part of Françoise's history was never to be broached. Spontaneously, like all children, Françoise had supported and helped her depressed mother without knowing the depression arose because she had never accepted the death of her own mother and little brother: she had never effectively mourned them.

When a tragic event is kept secret, it becomes like a phantom or ghost (in the psychoanalytical sense) for succeeding generations: an "opaque empty hole" that takes the place of a representation of the death of the grandmother and the little brother. This "phantom" interferes with the succession of generations, acting like a cyst that is unconsciously handed down from mother to daughter in the form of a family line disorder. The trauma in Françoise's past created a "freeze-frame" where the cyclical dimension of time gets jammed. Françoise's fibroma was reopening what happened to someone her age two generations earlier.

Repetition provides a way to understand and assimilate what happens in life. It is part of the human psyche. We have all been constructed from the energies interwoven out of the histories of both our family lines, and we hand down a state of being to our children which provides them with the foundations for their own structure. Thus, life repeats itself and since repetitive behaviour appears around the same age or around the same date as the original event, Anne Ancelin Schützenberger has conceptualized the phenomenon by naming it the "anniversary syndrome" (3).

Repetition is not always so clearly evident as in Françoise's case. But it is still puzzling to find that the same dates reappear for births, deaths, accidents, maladies and other significant events of life.

Symptoms generated by family line disorders

In this area, a woman's gynaecological problems, both functional and organic (4), always reflect impediments inherited from female ancestors. Gynaecological symptoms appear mainly in one of two ways. They may be linked with a woman's cycle: heaviness, pain, or bloating in the abdomen, breasts, or legs; irregular cycles; uterine bleeding; general exhaustion; moodiness, irritability, vulnerability and dissatisfaction. Alternatively, they may settle in: weight gain, especially in the breasts, abdomen or thighs; icy feet, hands and buttocks; non-malignant growths such as tumours, polyps, fibromas or cysts; or malignant ones such as cancer.

Whatever the symptoms, whether we have integrated the energies of our ancestors or are trying to escape them, these symptoms are always within us. If we do not become aware of them, we will remain unconsciously attached to them.

Most functional problems have been greatly reduced with the advent of contraceptive pills, because the pill puts the ovaries on hold. Since the pill's hormones replace those normally secreted by the ovaries, the synergetic connection between the pituitary gland and the ovaries is broken. Psychological and emotional disarray no longer influence the ovaries, which are temporarily put aside. Since the pill interrupts procreation and the succession of generations, women's health is less apt to fluctuate.

Women can regain their personal dynamism, instead of being held back by their inheritance from previous generations.

Nonetheless, intolerance to hormonal treatments is quite common. The pill's supplementary hormonal effects accentuate problems for these women. They feel like they are suffocating, imploding, unable to find a way out, unknowingly imprisoned in their family history.

Sterility and infertility

Problems of infertility where a woman gets pregnant but has repeated miscarriages and is unable to bring her pregnancy to term; infertile couples who cannot have a child although nothing is preventing them medically; or unwanted, unplanned pregnancies: all these problems are transgenerational. Their origin is ancestral.

With sterility, when examination finds everything normal, but no baby comes, there is certainly a blockage, but it is not physical. The woman ovulates, the man's sperm is fertile, the passages are clear in the fallopian tubes and the uterus: there is no physical obstacle to fertility. It can only be concluded that something else is in the way. The couple's desire is obviously present, but something is keeping them back, stopping them from changing from a boy and a girl into a father and a mother, stopping them from carrying forward their lineage. It can be very fruitful for such couples to engage in therapeutic work so they can move beyond the childhood status in which they have been imprisoned. Usually they do not know that the obstacle to their parenting plans comes from their respective family histories.

Unwanted pregnancies

With an unwanted pregnancy, it is as if a woman's body were directly connected to her mother's way of having children. The woman becomes pregnant at the age her mother got pregnant with her or with her brothers and sisters, or when her mother met a lover, or separated from the father of her children; in short, in all sorts of ways on the anniversary date of an event that marked her mother's life as a woman. Being pregnant in this case expresses a genealogical repetition and she may try to rid herself of this by having an abortion so as to be born to herself.

Unwanted pregnancies are never inconsequential. But, contrary to popular belief, they do not always represent the unconscious desire for a child. It is important to understand what is happening. While the desire to be a mother in the future is not called into question, this particular pregnancy is not consonant with a desire to share parenthood with a man. The woman is caught up alone between herself and her past, and so is the man. They discover that they are not infertile, but they have not made a child together.

Either the woman senses this, she is not unhappy, she did not want this child, so she is confronted with the fact that she made this happen to her body so that she could grow up. She was careless with her contraception. Or else, she is sad and unhappy, in which case she needs to realize that her sadness is not because her child will not be born, but because of the feelings involved in separating herself from her maternal lineage. In such a case, the genealogical search is the same as for painful periods: we need to investigate the heritage handed down by the women who preceded us, focusing on illnesses, mourning of losses, how their children were conceived, as well as repeated dates.

Didier Dumas conceptualized this idea with the term "the maternal unthought" (5), meaning not so much the way in which our mother has impeded us as the way in which she was herself somatically impeded by her inherited trauma.

The importance of knowing one's genealogy

Every tradition tells us that we inherit from our ancestors. They hand down their strengths and their weaknesses, and the latter can manifest as physical or psychological maladies. Maladies of ancestral origin, these family line disorders, can "possess" us, becoming recurrent or chronic. I believe that to set ourselves loose it is indispensable to acquaint ourselves with our transgenerational history. This after all is the terrain in which disorders appear.

To consider the transgenerational aspect of our existence takes us to the universal dimension of life. Our children extend us forward while turning us into future ancestors as parents, grandparents, great-grandparents. Since death is inseparable from life, we are born into the succession of generations in a particular position where we receive the inheritance from our ancestors and pass on that inheritance to our children and our grandchildren. By living, we automatically carry forward knowledge and traditions. This human condition is recognized by peoples who practice ancestor worship. In our culture, our relationship with our ancestors may be conscious or unconscious. And it is the unconscious which is at work in symptoms.

Life is a continuous, cyclical process and death is part of that. Adults bring children into the world and accompany their parents to their death. Death, meaning the emptiness created by the loss of a loved one (6), is no longer perceived as a personal tragedy. It becomes normal for "the elderly" to leave us: they have lived their lives, in their own way. It is important to respect them, accompany them to the end, and say goodbye to them both to support them and to come to terms with their departure from life.

Of course, this will not prevent the sorrow and distress of no longer being able to have a loved one near. But instead of being held captive and paralyzed by suffering, one can place death in a larger context, and so perceive it differently.

When a younger person dies prematurely in an accident or from illness, the normal and natural element in the inescapable passage from life to death is missing. Yet transgenerational psychoanalysis shows us that a premature death is not necessarily

88

purely coincidental. Sometimes such a death can be explained as a process of repetition of a date, an age, a geographical area, a hidden or unknown tragedy. A brother or sister dying at the same age as an ancestor, mothers dying in childbirth, neonatal deaths, suicide, cancer and many other illnesses, war victims, genocides.

The importance of ancestral memory has declined in our civilization. Since we no longer have beliefs, rituals or myths that refer to ancestral memory, creating our family tree is a way of investigating how our ancestors lived. To discover it, guided by the awareness of what we need to know, is to recognize the place allotted to us. It is not just a matter of satisfying a curiosity but of making contact with those who came before you, thanks to whom we are alive now. How did they live? Did they appreciate their life, or did they remain isolated behind their walls? Were they depressed, violent, unhappy as children? Were they hustlers, adventurers or creators, or did they repeat their family history? As we gradually build our family trees, we discover the origins of our repetitive behaviour, obstacles, failures, fears and illnesses. We also discover the origins of our talents, capacities and skills.

The effects of building a genosociogram

Putting together a genosociogram enables us to connect with the energy of our ancestors. It is a tool to put things back in order. We reclaim our personal history. We have a larger picture since parents and ancestors have their own way of looking at things, their own truth, and we learn to think of them in *our* own way. Placing our ancestors in the context of their lives allows us to understand them, to realize that they too had a history and to dissolve any resentments or idealizations. It's not about separating ourselves from them but seeing how we are an extension of them. By accepting them as they were, we can take up our rightful place. Researching our genosociogram allows us to accept our past and to free ourselves from the unspoken truths, the omissions or the lies in our family myths.

Creating our family tree honours our ancestors by bringing them back into existence. It begins with a search for information from parents and grandparents and those close to them, but also in official records. This search is an opportunity to encounter people we have never known, to discover the conditions in which they were conceived, the world in which they grew up, how they lived their lives as men, women, fathers, mothers, sisters or brothers, and about their lawful or unlawful love affairs. Whatever their story, we are able to form a representation of these ancestors and of the energies they incarnated and carried forward. By making them come alive, we release the forces locked inside secrets or ignorance. By making sense of their history, we re-establish a connection, communication and flexibility.

The connection is restored, casting light on our own makeup. A genosociogram frees us from the unconscious ties that kept us in bondage. It provides the energy that drives us to construct ourselves and forge ahead. Becoming oneself is not a betrayal or an abandonment of our ancestors. On the contrary, it affirms that what they gave us has allowed us to become what we are. They can rest in peace, happy and content.

Life pushes us forward, and we need not wait for the people in our family to drive us. Had they been capable of doing it, they would have done so already. When we establish our family tree, what is at issue is not whether we love our ancestors or have a grudge against them, but rather that we recognize what they were. Our ancestors are our foundation, our base. We rediscover them so as to say goodbye to them. They will no longer need to absorb our attention. With the energy we acquire, we enlarge and consolidate our base, which will not just allow but will compel us to go forward and create our own life. In this way, we prolong our ancestors without being dependent on them. A genosociogram is not only an act of separation but also an act of "extension."

Without doing the work of tracing their genealogy, men and women have a strong tendency to adopt or protect the "official family myth," perpetuating the suffering, illness, lies, denial and failures that are carried down the family line. What happens in this case? Because we are constituted from a lie, transmission becomes blurred, the truth gets lost, and we find ourselves cut off from the ties that anchor us to our ancestors. If we cannot know our true history, we float without bearings, with no base or support from which to build ourselves. Yet the truth, though we remain ignorant of it, will still come out in one way or another, and act in its own name. In life, that will produce repetitive phenomena through which the past seeks to make itself heard.

These repetitive phenomena appear when, instead of acting according to our own ideas and personal desires, our actions unconsciously are driven by these "phantom" energy structures that turn a person into "Dr Jekyll and Mr Hyde." This is so because we construct ourselves by duplicating the familial and social characteristics of our parents. This assimilation happens unconsciously, so if we are not wary, they can take control of our lives.

Our cellular memory is made up of our ancestral heritage. Duplication is a physiological process that allows this heritage to be handed down from generation to generation. Wanting to escape it is an illusion. If we try to run from our heritage, we only give it more energy and make it stronger. To get away from these repetitions, the first step is to recognize them, accept them and stop clashing futilely with them. Though we did indeed construct ourselves out of this heritage, we now need to leave it behind, to stop indulging it, so as to be free to add our "personal touch" and construct a personality that is really our own.

If our intention is genuine, becoming aware of how we are imitating our forebears, unconsciously identifying with them, is the first step towards change and transformation. Mathilde, who I advised to draw up her genosociogram, became aware of this in the following dream: "It was at a family banquet. I found myself among my paternal and maternal ancestors, very few of whom I knew. There was a warm atmosphere of reunion, which gave me an incredible inner strength and joy. But as time went on, I began to feel oppressed, feverish, lonely and stifled. To my amazement, I saw I was attached to my ancestors with chains, and, even more amazing, I was the one holding the chains."

Certainly, with gynaecological disorders, the first thing to investigate is our maternal heritage. But we also need to see how both of our hereditary lines are involved. Our paternal grandmother also influences our femininity and who we are. As Didier Dumas explained in *L'Ange et le Fantôme*, what is handed down from one generation to the next are the phantoms, carried by each parent, that have similarities or complementarities with one another. So, it is important that a woman does not neglect to investigate her paternal lineage. After all, don't we say, "They have come together for better or for worse?" In the case of Françoise's fibroma, learning that her father's place in his family was in between two dead brothers helped Françoise to realize why he could not help his wife and his daughters release themselves from the death of their grandmother and little brother.

Care

With this kind of pathology, as I see it, the repair work is two-dimensional in the sense that it involves two different parts of ourselves: restoring our "vertical axis" based on what we come to understand about our ancestors, and doing therapeutic energy work on our "horizontal axis" to heal our bodies.

Discovering that her grandmother died at age forty-three allowed Françoise to make sense of her own fibroma and her female relatives' hysterectomies. Learning the circumstances of her grandmother's death helped her to realize that this grandmother had her own past, that she, too, had carried a "phantom" within her from generations further back, and that was why she died. This kind of discovery re-establishes a link in the succession of generations.

Françoise's energy therapy aimed to bring life back to her uterus, which had frozen up and lost its elasticity because it had been deprived of the nourishing energy absorbed by the "phantom grandmother." Françoise's uterus had grown larger and was bleeding. It had become detrimentally hyperactive, but in a way that was so surreptitious and deeply buried that Françoise could not feel it. Instead of resting, as it should have since Françoise was not pregnant, it was active and enlarged, evidence of undesirable excess energy.

According to Chinese medicine, in a case like this the uterus is disrupted by "perverse energy" (7) that activates it, without one realizing it. Treatment involves bringing fresh energy to the pelvis, the uterus, the ovaries and their connections to other parts of the body. By asking Françoise to focus her attention on her uterus and to feel energy flowing through it, I taught her to re-energize her pelvis. That way, she could truly integrate it into herself, as something alive that no longer belonged to her grandmothers or her great-grandmothers.

To be healthy, we need to nurture our authentic selves. By discovering and acting in accordance with what is good for us, we break the cycle of repetition. Without this therapeutic work on our family history, we may remain, like many women, reliant on family secrets that date from before we were born: licit or illicit love affairs, questions of honour, tragedies, ill-nesses or failed mourning that were not resolved by prior generations. If we are not wary, if we do not pay attention to the way problems sound the alarm, and if we refuse to examine how transgenerational repetition structures our lives, for better or for worse, we risk even more damage.

By not acknowledging that this is the nature of life, we run the risk of being brought back into line by the invisible but relentless law of the succession of generations. This is what we are talking about when we say, "She died of the same disease as her mother." Even though science does not know how the code is handed down, we do know the energy it carries is very powerful. In the last three generations, women's lives have changed radically. But the ancestral habit of saying nothing about problems of sexuality and death, of keeping them secret, is still alive and kicking.

"He visits the iniquity of the fathers upon their children to the third and fourth generation" biblically translates our dependence on our ancestral heritage since the dawn of time.

Notes

1. The idea of the tomb and the phantom, or ghost, was developed at the beginning of the 1970s by the psychoanalysts Nicolas Abraham and Maria Torok. See Nicolas Abraham and Maria Torok, *L'Ecorce et le Noyau* (Paris: Flammarion, 1999).
2. See Marie Cardinal, *Les mots pour le dire*. Paris: Grasset, 1976. Translated as *The Words to Say It* (Cambridge, MA: VanVactor & Goodheart, 1983).
3. Anne Ancelin Schützenberger, *Aïe, mes aïeux! op. cit.*
4. A *functional problem* is an imbalance that has not been ingrained in the physical body. The organs involved look normal under examination, but they do not function properly. With an *organic problem*, the organ is observably affected with a cyst, a fibroma or a cancer.
5. Didier Dumas, *L'Ange et le Fântome op. cit.*
6. See Aude Zeller, *À l'épreuve de la vieillesse* (Paris, Desclée de Brouwer, 2003).
7. In this case, "perverse" means "going in the wrong direction." Chinese medicine distinguishes many types of energy: nutritive and protective energy, which take care of the body and its organs, and perverse energy, which interferes and creates disorders.

CHAPTER SIX

Desire

"Why am I still having such a hard time with men?" asked Anne, aged thirty-five. "I know how to be seductive, how to make myself beautiful, how to dance, but I don't know how to desire a man, and I don't know what to do with a man's desire for me. When a man desires me, I blush and turn away. I want to run, even though deep down I'm dying to say 'yes' to him. I was taught to want to be a mother and to want a satisfying job, but nobody ever taught me how to feel desire for a man I love, or how to joyfully welcome his desire for me."

In my practice I see women who are young and not so young, with or without a man in their life, married, living with someone, divorced, alone, students, mothers, retirees. Many ask me for help with the same problem. They want to know how to live out their femininity: to be glad to be a woman, to be desirable and to feel desire.

Despite appearing to be liberated, women are still the receptacles of feminine transmissions that split them in two in two different ways. First, they are cut off from communicating freely with men. It is not that they don't desire men, but an invisible curtain woven of taboos, shame, guilt, ignorance, and lack of self-confidence envelops them in a fog that separates them from men and prevents them from expressing themselves freely. They go to pieces under the effect their emotions. They no longer know how to listen to men or how to talk to them. Not even daring to look at men, they remain petrified and mute, or else they get suddenly agitated and talk about whatever comes into their head, everything except what they want to say. It is as if their desire made them panic.

The second way they are cut off is in their energy. This is a true divide, with their whole being separated into two: the top separated from the bottom, the body from spirit, thought from heart, heart from sex, thought from desire. These women are unable to feel whole. They have not been able to fully take possession of themselves, nor to create unity between the thoughts in their head, the feelings in their heart, and the sensations in their genitals. They are unable to experience their sexuality as they would wish, and when they are with a man, they fail to achieve the fulfilment they have been waiting for.

Inherited social and cultural burdens

In the time of our grandmothers and great-grandmothers, sexuality for pleasure was taboo: it was a sin of the flesh. It existed in brothels, in exchange for money, or else it was only known to women of "easy virtue," considered as whores. Our grandmothers were "as pure as the driven snow," innocent and ignorant. They had never been prepared to think about their own genitals, let alone a man's. Nobody ever told them about their future life as a woman.

Since their mothers, grandmothers and aunts had shrouded sexuality in mysterious whispers that were not for the ears of young girls, new brides had no idea what would happen to them on their wedding night. They were obliged to remain virgins, not just physically but also mentally. All they could imagine about the future was that they would have children. When it came to marriage, they were assailed by every imaginable fear.

They could only hope that their husband would inform them about that nameless thing, sex. Everything was in his hands. But most of the time, the husband remained silent. He did not have the words to speak about his own sexuality let alone his wife's. It was claimed that silence was a form of respect for his bride, since the only words available for talking about sexuality were crude and vulgar.

First change: women think (1945)

The First World War decimated the male population, putting women in the workplace. They had lost their husbands, brothers and fathers, and began to contemplate taking care of themselves, managing their assets, doing paid work in order to finance the household and raise the children.

French women had to wait until April 1945 before they were given the right to vote and regarded as citizens. Henceforth they were recognized as able to have a view, an opinion about the political and social life of the country: women could "think."

It was a radical upheaval and the first transformation that gave women the right to exist in ways other than through maternity. From then on, they enthusiastically set to work to build this new, gender-mixed society.

Second change: birth control (1965)

Twenty years later, in the mid nineteen sixties, a new "bombshell" exploded: the contraceptive pill. The great majority of women welcomed it favourably, happy and relieved to be able to choose whether or not to have children. They now had the chance to be independent. They wanted to take their place in society, not be equated solely with the maternal function, but were still willing to look after the children to whom they did give birth. This second transformation was to radically change the lives of men and women. Contraception has put humanity in control of its desire to have children, although not absolute control since we do not entirely understand the mystery of life. But contraception has raised the question of our reproduction, the desire to extend our lineage and to become a parent.

Contraception frees us from subordination to the body's biology. We can now choose to bring children into the world when there is a conscious, shared desire in both parents. The pill allows us to take responsibility for bringing our descendants into the world instead of being subjected to them. In our great-grandmothers' day, sexuality was most often a matter relating to the body, to biology, for the purposes of reproduction. With the pill, sexuality has become a matter of human encounters and of desire, allowing the mental and spiritual dimensions to move to the forefront.

When two consenting adults want a child together, that child is projected into a very different world than the one that child would have entered if s/he were unplanned. This shared desire means the child is welcomed into a favourable, reassuring matrix, already firmly rooted in her/his parents' shared story. It gives the child the power to enjoy life and self-actualize. Conversely, an unplanned child is the fruit of a meeting of two unconsciouses, not of two persons. Such a child risks feeling rootless. This lack of early parental recognition may keep the child from finding the internal stability to construct her/his social and sexual identity.

Third change: sexual liberation?

The advent of the contraceptive pill gave rise to the idea that women's sexual fulfilment—and by extension that of men with women—would come about automatically. The women of my generation thought that, unlike their mothers, their lives would no longer be conditioned by the risk of getting pregnant, which until then had constrained sexuality. They would—or so it was thought—be able to discover sexual fulfilment and finally experience what had always been denied them. With the pill, the taboo against sexuality was gone. We were consenting adults. We were in luck.

This third transformation gave rise to the sexual revolution of the 1970s. It was a euphoric time: from then on, liberated sexuality would be part of our life; we would be able to explore it. We could get to know a future husband physically without making a permanent commitment. We could choose the father of our children without having to marry him. In the 1970s, 30% of children in France were conceived by couples who lived together but were not married (1). *Coitus interruptus* was no longer necessary: men were delighted, and women believed this would help them reach orgasm. They thought that if only a man could climax inside them without fear, they would automatically follow suit. The assumption that male ejaculation necessarily led to female orgasm was widespread.

At that time, men and women began to speak to each other about sexuality. Couples began to talk to each other about themselves, about their past and about their intimacy. Men and women tried to establish new patterns of behaviour and to recognize the position of sexuality. Before contraception, according to the social mores of the time, to deserve respect a woman had to be a virgin, "pure" and "intact" when she married. It was still acceptable for marriage to be arranged by the family. Later on, love became the main criterion: "I will choose and marry the man I love." With contraception and women's financial independence, the next stage was reached: marriage itself could be called into question, in favour of a moral commitment to love, to be true to one's word, and have confidence in one's own heart.

This social and sexual revolution allowed women to become full-fledged "thinking female beings" who dared to speak out and express themselves. In social activities they flourished and became accomplished, securing a hard-won position at the workplace. Men recognized their efficiency and granted them equality, although this has still not been achieved everywhere. A great battle had been won, but what has become of women's femininity today? Two generations after the advent of contraception, have women really taken charge of their own sexuality?

Parental fulfilment

Nowadays, parenthood has undeniably made progress. Motherhood and fatherhood have flourished, to the child's benefit. Not only is a baby a person in his/her own right, but so is the foetus (2). With haptonomy, the science of emotional contact founded by Franz Veldman, men are active participants in the gestation of their child. In some maternity hospitals, discussion groups are held where expectant fathers can learn their new role. They may also be present during labour and delivery, so that giving birth is no longer the preserve of women but a place where a couple welcomes their child together. New fathers actively take part in raising their child, with as much pleasure whether it is a girl or a boy.

Continued ignorance about sexuality

The twenty-first century woman thinks, reacts and lives very differently from her grandmothers and great-grandmothers. But even though she occupies a new place in society, she still carries within her the models of women in her family, by ignoring the festive, regenerating and structuring role of sexuality.

This series of changes still do not entail harmony between being a woman and being a mother. Originally, contraception was a social transformation that limited the number of births. It brought to light the fact that being a mother and being a woman were two separate functions, which do not belong to the same space-time. But to be able to accomplish a fulfilling sexuality, social change and medical development are not enough. Of course, these developments are necessary to "set the tone," but more work is needed to learn the music. The music of sexual pleasure is handed down individually and through the family. From that heritage, each one of us puts her own words to the erotic melody.

Desire: the energy that makes the encounter possible

Sexual desire is a force that drives you towards the unknown, towards difference and towards novelty, in the hope of becoming complete. For a woman, expressing her sexual desire means showing a man the "vibes" she feels for him. It means knowing how to respond to the glance of someone who is really looking at her, to words that make her laugh or that touch and permeate her triggering an emotion or sensation that foreshadows the pleasure of penetration.

When a woman expresses her desire, a man knows his presence makes her feel something that has specifically to do with who he is: a sensation in her body or an emotion in her heart. He attracts us, gives us confidence, impassions us. In short, we are interested and relate. There is no single way to make this interest known. Each woman has her own style, her originality or her little tricks for expressing her desire.

The expression of desire creates a tension that motivates us and makes us want to advance further to test whether the initial perception at the first meeting persists. The future beckons us and forces us to move. To embrace our desire releases energy that would otherwise remain locked in fantasy. It means no longer saying "no" to someone else so that you can say "yes" to yourself. Making known your desire means starting out on your own path and taking the risk of opening yourself to the unknown. Women have often told me they do not dare show their interest because they are afraid of being disappointed. Disappointed by what? By a negative reaction? Better to take the risk of being alive than to remain stuck in the dreams of an asexual young girl!

Of course, if that desire cannot be reciprocated, it is important not to go on dreaming of an impossible outcome. Being aware of that will set us free to meet someone new. Young girls' dreams are filled with suitors who carry them off so they do not have to decide for themselves. This attitude is a mixture of the fear of leaving "mummy" and the desire for a man to winkle us away from her. It sometimes results in the woman letting herself be seduced without feeling any genuine desire. If, on the contrary, we are active in our desire, if we acknowledge and enact it, we will allow love to reach another level: the space of possibility, of a true encounter, of knowledge that permits us to open ourselves to pleasure.

When desire is inhibited

But even though today our choice and free will should help when it comes to love, most women still find themselves caught up in emotional dramas with the man they love. As soon as they are out of their social context or their maternal role and find themselves in the intimate realm with a man, it is disastrous. A new feminine order has yet to be built. Faced with a man's desire, women do not know how to open themselves either to his desire or to their own. Either they want him to take care of them and be in charge of everything, or they want to run away, withdrawing into themselves or keeping away from any emotional involvement. They find themselves just as inhibited as their grandmothers and their great-grandmothers.

Some women have successfully ventured into living their desire and discovering a pleasurable and fulfilling sexual life, thanks to the liberated mores of our time, open-minded families and supportive girlfriends. But when they meet a man and really fall in love, that is when their heart and soul are involved, when the question of commitment, of living together, of marriage arises, or most often when a child is born, things go awry. These women regress. The feminine model of their female ancestors automatically comes to the fore and takes over. Unknowingly, they follow in the footsteps of their ancestors, although that model is no longer relevant. They notice that their desire is gone. It has vanished, and their openness to the desire of the one they love has gone too.

In the long run, if this state of affairs persists, they are no longer even sure whether they love this man. The sexuality which they so wholeheartedly claimed and defended fades away, and maternal asexuality takes over. They end up being like their mothers: energetically cut in half.

Many more women than we think live with no sexuality at all. These women have constructed themselves in the absence of any new verbalization and have unconsciously duplicated the sexual model their mother gave them, like one Russian doll fits inside another. Whether they are young or not so young, for them desire for a man does not exist. Basically, they do not like men: they may love them as fathers or as brothers but not their masculinity. "Sexuality isn't for me. It doesn't interest me," as Nathalie's mother said.

Most women's experience of sexuality, one way or another, is unsatisfying. They feel desire but never experience regenerative pleasure inside their body. Frustrated, they are denied access to sexual fulfilment. Such women may love a man with their mind and heart, but not with their body.

"All the same," Mélanie told me, "I love this man. He's attractive, I appreciate his qualities, I think about him, I'm attentive, and I give him presents he likes. I'm happy I met him. There's joy and understanding between us. And lots of tenderness. We like each other's bodies. Our kisses are delicious. But as soon as there's penetration, my feeling of pleasure becomes insignificant compared to the intensity I feel when he caresses my vulva and clitoris in foreplay."

Mélanie's body was letting her know it was still configured in the "little girl" mode rather than as a woman. When she was a child, Mélanie's body was unable to build itself in such a manner as to hear the call of penetration. It only knew how to deal with the preliminaries of lovemaking. For Mélanie's body, penetration was either bland or painful. Her genitals had not reached maturity.

Mélanie went on, "I love his penis inside me—or rather, I love the idea of his penis being inside me. But basically I don't love his genitals. They bother me. I don't know what to do with them. When I'm faced with them, I'm powerless. They are strangers. I don't know what they are. They have to get on without me. My inside is an abstraction to me. It's not that I feel nothing, but I expect his genitals to awaken mine."

Much as Melanie loved the man with whom she lived, she did not know she could desire his genitals, long for them, appreciate them, call them to her, welcoming, celebrating them and letting herself be overcome by their energy and power.

Every possible kind of problem with penetration exists: from penetration being a total impossibility, painful penetration, total lack of feeling in the vagina, to the eroticization of the openings of the mouth and the anus so that sodomy and fellatio are preferred, with no call from the vagina to be penetrated. These are the most common patterns I come across among my patients. They continue to suffer from ignorance and taboos that prevent them from experiencing pleasure inside their body.

Because the only bodily construction they were entitled to in infancy was that of being breastfed and caressed, their sexuality is stuck at the foreplay stage of lovemaking. They love with their hearts and their minds, but they remain very passive sexually and disinclined to express their desires. They did not know how to embark on the discovery of pleasure for its own sake, although their minds are full of those dreams. To avoid betraying their mother, they remain "virgins" by remaining their mother's daughters in the kingdom of childhood.

For these women, dissatisfaction sets in with time. They lose hope that their sexuality might change, and they hide a broken heart. Little by little, unspoken anxiety takes the place of joy. What they need to understand at this point is that they love their man like they loved their mother. As little girls, they could conceive neither of their father's genitals nor of what their mother did with them. They were not given a functioning image either of a man's genitals or of their own, or of what the two could do together.

Such is the "sexual gynaecology" that these women have helped me create. They include, as we saw, Therese and her husband, Nathalie and her thrush, Catherine and her cystitis, Anne and her desire, but also the slipped disc that severed Françoise's energetic structure between the top and the bottom so she was unable to move. For these women to recover, they needed to restore and consolidate the energy flow that keeps us upright and make us feel we are women.

The body is not invaginated

In all these cases, while the sharing of ideas and of the heart allowed these women to love a man, their experience of having a female body was not "invaginated," which means that the idea of their vagina as a cavity that beckons from the inside had never come to be represented as part of their body image; the cavity that beckons from the inside had not been constituted. Such a body remains impenetrable, like that of a little girl who could never imagine what role a man's genitals might play in the pleasure of being a woman. Penetration could not be established as the path to discovering and exploring an interior journey—let alone a breach leading into eternity.

Misunderstanding the energetic dimension of sexuality makes it seem purely mechanical. Instead of uniting two energetic bodies, the genitals are unaware of how to exchange their vibratory powers. Their contact becomes irritating. It may heat or burn the vulva or anaesthetize the vulva when the woman goes absent from herself. The resulting frustration is serious and dangerous, placing both the man's and the woman's body in a "pressure cooker," or worse, in a tomb. This claustration causes inertia and hysteria in women, and apathy and violence in men.

In any case, a man's desire to make love is not just a desire to make love with an attentive, respectful woman whom he loves. It is also a desire to make love with a woman who desires him and wants to make love with him.

How to break the cycle of transgenerational repetition

In all the cases described above, the women are unaware of being psychologically imprisoned within their maternal lineage. This imprisonment becomes most strikingly obvious with the birth of a child. A new mother is even less aware of this, because her child really needs her, and she is absorbed by the reality of that need. It does not bother her that she no longer wants to make love, because her child has made her complete and she still loves her man. She doesn't feel anything is missing. Most of the time, she wants only one thing: to feel less tired, to restore her vitality in the arms of her child's father through a moment of shared celebration of their new state of parenthood.

However, if this situation persists, the mother will find herself exhausted—and so will the father. Partly because she never stops for one second, but also because she is within her mother's energetic structure rather than her own and does not know how to regenerate herself. The bond that connects her to her child and to her man is a bond of love, of heart and soul, but by itself it does not re-energize the physical body.

To remedy this form of transgenerational repetition, first of all one must be aware of it. Any change implies learning, which it is important to take seriously, to set aside time for it. It involves the reconstructive work whereby new imprints and memories are ingrained within the self to supplant those that have been carried for decades. For the woman, the first task is to recognize and accept her inability to construct herself as a woman who feels desire so as to make room for a new self-image.

This requires a change in state of mind, rethinking how one's sexuality functions, so as to create a different life from the one that was handed down. It is a task of rebirth that must be reimagined and maintained every day in order to incorporate our genitals so that they become part of our entire being. By constantly renewing the intention of bringing life to our genitals and integrating them into our body image, new imprints can gradually be registered. This occurs through sensory awareness—that is, through the sensations we feel when we think about it. To make our genitals part of us, we simply need to think about them and be aware of what we feel in doing so. This way, we create the sensory skin that should have been developed as a young girl. Experiencing this new dimension of desire uncovers unknown sensations. The pleasure so derived signals that these have a structuring effect on our organism. This is the healing effect of therapeutic work. It shows us that the power we have over our body is such that we can change and remodel it. Refining the sensations, we feel, as much in daily life as during sexual activity, shows the way to reconstruction.

Knowing that our female body is "invaginated," that it has a cavity, that we need to joyfully make room inside to receive a man's penis and the energy it carries means we must learn to think about the place of sexuality in our lives in a completely different way from what was handed down to us. It means accepting that we are glad and proud that this meeting takes place inside our bodies and knowing how to appreciate the difference and the complementarity of the two sexes.

These are the new imprints that we can hand down to our future daughters, so they can learn to be women who feel desire and know how to welcome and receive a man's desire.

"But," Patricia wanted to know, "does that mean that women will know how to be women only if their mothers felt good about themselves, are able to talk to their daughters and cherish the value of pleasure?"

Ideally of course we should have parents who desire each other and know how to enjoy that. In that case, a daughter constructs herself by identifying sexually with her mother. As an adult, she will not encounter all these obstacles to fully experiencing and expressing her sexual desires. But people raised like this are few and far between. Most women today have to admit they belong to a pivotal generation caught between a repressive past and a future that is still in the making. It is important that mothers are able to speak authentically to their daughters about their own sexuality, because in any case sexuality is something that is handed down.

"I took me a long time to discover sexual pleasure, even after I began taking the pill. You know what I mean: your grandmother couldn't teach me a thing. But you belong to a generation that allows you to know that pleasure is something you can open yourself to and experience." Unless her mother talks to her like that, how is a daughter to know that her mother, who freely mentions tampons and contraceptive pills, did not know the first thing about lovemaking and has remained an inhibited little girl? Realizing and accepting that her own mother lived in sexual ignorance takes a long time.

If, on the other hand, a mother can explain what she had to learn in order to change, her daughter will feel free to do better than her mother and will venture beyond to discover sexuality for herself. A mother who has never experienced fulfilment should talk about this too. She could say to her daughter, "Don't be like me! I knew nothing at all. I was always expecting it to happen out of the blue, but it never did. It was very late when I found out that lovemaking has to be learned. You are aware of that, so you're bound to do better than I did." If a mother propels her daughter towards womanhood in this way, the daughter will know that she can create her own life as a woman, and that she has permission to learn and to change.

In summary, down through the generations, from our great-grandmothers through our grandmothers to our mothers, women's functioning has shifted from passivity and total dependence on a mother and on a husband to a freedom, which, still today, has yet to be fully achieved.

There has been real progress, but if I think back over the thirty years that I have been listening to women, I have to admit they still have great difficulty taking control of their emotional and sexual lives. In actual fact, women's liberation has been essentially social. It is on that level that they have radically succeeded in differentiating themselves from their grandmothers and great-grandmothers. In this way, they more actively exist in their masculine dimension becoming autonomous and creative. But their feminine side remains nested in their female lineage and they lack the secure base that would let them express their sexual desire or respond to the sexual desire of a man. Being cut off in this way makes for anguish and a lack of self-esteem. Often, they lock themselves up in this dissatisfaction of their life as women, not knowing how to take advantage of the love men can bring them.

The starting point of a man's sexual desire is the genitals, while a woman's is in her heart, between her two breasts

Women often say, "I need a lot of time," complaining about how men want to get to penetration so quickly. Chinese sexology taught me that men and women are made differently and that a whole tactical sequence and a game must be devised for the genitals to match up with each other and come together at the right moment.

A man's sexual arousal goes straight to his penis, while a woman's begins at her breasts and in her heart, and then travels downwards to her genitals. This explains the mismatch between a man's frequently immediate desire for penetration and a woman's desire, which needs time for the energy in her heart to move to her genitals. The creativity of the erotic courtship enables lovers to "adjust" to each other, to bring their desires into unison. Confidence allows the body to give itself over to the pleasure of the dance. Creativity in lovemaking becomes more finely tuned when each partner can put into words what they want and expect. So, by each knowing themselves and their partner, their coming together can not only unfold and renew itself, but also evolve over time and with experience. Clearly, for the wonder of the encounter to take place, penetration should occur when a woman wants it and when she is ready. But very often, without her even realizing it, the energy of a woman's genitals remains impervious to receiving the penis.

When a woman is attracted to a man, she always begins with dreaming about him. That is what awakens her senses. She is attracted to him, but if she is split in two she does not always feel her genitals as willing to open for him. The energy of her desire and her thoughts, even if they move through her heart, do not get as far as her genitals. There is no downward motion.

A man's sexual desire starts in his body, in his muscles. He needs to respond to the physical tension that this desire brings about in his genitals. When he has an erection, he is stirred by the desire to thrust his penis inside the body of the woman, and once penetration occurs, he feels his penis is in its rightful place. It makes him feel whole, in the true sense of the word, because his entire body is suffused and flooded. He feels that he exists. His sexual energy starts in his genitals and rises to his heart and his head. For him, a woman's body is a place where he can anchor himself to the earth and be regenerated. The quality of the relationship is what touches his heart, enhances his life and drives his thoughts.

For a woman, desire is a force that encourages her to seek out a man, that urges her to satisfy her curiosity, and go towards what is unknown to her. It means accepting and welcoming the regenerative unknown that he carries, and which will sustain her. It is a "heavenly elevator" that lifts her up.

Woman and their desire: floating heads

For generations, there has been a big difference in what is handed down to girls and what is handed down to boys. The principal difference is that from the beginning a boy knows he will have a sexual life of pleasure when he grows up. He does not know how, because he has been given no explanations to help him think about it, but he knows it—his spirit knows it. Generally, a girl knows no such thing. Because she receives no sexual education, the spirit of the girl—and of the future woman—remains separate from her genitals. Since the two are not connected, the spirit does not know how to stir and open her genitals. Therefore, the genitals remain blocked or kept apart, and when a woman falls in love, she is inhibited by all sorts of taboos that either keep her from the man she loves or drive him away completely. Most women are "female torsos," whose life stops at the waist—or, to be more precise, at the diaphragm. They are "floating heads" on top of a disembodied body.

Something else that needs to be understood is that it is through the co-penetration of the genitals—anatomically inside the vagina but energetically in the uterus—that both man and woman find their place. The uterus is designed not just for reproduction. It is also the energy matrix for the woman's own construction and that of her partner. It is central to a woman's orgasm, the alchemical crucible where masculine and feminine energies meet. In the uterus, the sexual forces come together and seek unison to enhance each other's potential to the fullest. It is where each partner is ultimately acknowledged.

So, what is desire?

Desire is a form of tension that, by definition, tends towards novelty, towards what is farthest and highest, towards the unknown, in the hope of self-realization, of finding completeness. The tension of desire both beckons and propels us forward. It is possessed and contained by our spirit.

If there is no prospect of discovery, we remain within sameness. Nothing beckons and desire does not emerge.

In the loving encounter of the flesh, only desire can call forth a rich and satisfying sexuality, because pleasure is the realization of desire. Pleasure consists in seizing a morsel of the future in the present, something hoped for or which seems to have fallen out of the blue, embedding itself in the body in the form of delicious sensations.

Desire is what makes life sparkle. It is the prime mover in life. At birth, it is the desire to live; later in childhood, it is the desire to grow; with adolescence, it is the desire to realize oneself, to become oneself in harmony with our own and our partner's genitals. Desire opens the door to the future: "What is it that I want? What do I wish for?" It makes us ask ourselves those questions: it makes us independent. It is behind our conscious and unconscious choices. It determines the directions we take and the paths we follow. It allows us to be unique while being connected to the community. Desire is our guide in accomplishing our life.

Notes

1. See Évelyne Sullerot, *Quels pères? Quels fils?* (Paris: Fayard, 1992) and Didier Dumas, *Sans père et sans parole: La place du père dans l'équilibre de l'enfant* (Paris: Hachette Littératures, 1999).
2. See Jean-Marie Delassus, *Le Génie du fœtus: Vie prénatale et origine de l'homme* (Paris: Dunod, 2001).

CHAPTER SEVEN

What is making love?

When we make love, what happens to us is not part of everyday life—it is extraordinary. A new sensuality reveals itself. We are moving toward the discovery and creation of a new sensory skin—building it as we discover it. We need to pass through these sensations to feel the desire to caress and to be caressed.

As infants and children, we need caresses and human warmth so that we can construct ourselves and grow. As adults, we still need human warmth. Lovemaking is the time to be lovingly touched, inside and out. Receiving love and caresses is obviously vital to the infant.

In adult sexuality, caresses create a space for exchange, where each partner is present to him/herself and to the other. It is a mutual caress, which each one simultaneously gives to and receives from the other, producing a sensation that takes us from the outside to the inside of our bodies. It is the entrance to the world of lovemaking. It is a dance in which both partners must adjust to each other and synchronize. This is something they both do together, not just one or the other alone. The vibratory world of sensations and images harks back to our experience as a baby, before knowing how to speak. Discovering, inhabiting, and exploring that world enables us to experience, individually and together, a journey comprising different stages.

Courtship displays

The amorous display includes everything that happens before two bodies touch. It is a transitional space that lets you temporarily set aside your usual, mundane habits of acting and thinking for a while, so as to enter another scene where the focus is on other perceptions of your body. These are perceptions that pertain to the imagination and the vibratory waves of our sensuality whereby our desire for union is expressed.

Each partner needs to feel flattered to have been chosen by the other and happy to confirm that the other has made a good choice. This is the moment when each says "yes" to a promised coming together of their bodies, and each is willing to involve their genitals in their life with this special person. Both partners show how attractive they find the other in their own creative way, and that they are ready to venture into the world of sensual pleasure together.

This is when we give ourselves time to create a shared space, before the encounter of the genitals. It can be a time for walks where we together admire a beautiful landscape; a time for sustained, penetrating gazes; or for bursts of shared laughter and smiles that bring us very close. It can be a time for words that caress the ears and for movements that bring two bodies into tune. Dancers and musicians at the same time, we connect to "get in tune" with each other before improvising the duet about to be played.

Creating a shared space: foreplay and the encounter between the genitals

Now come the caresses and kisses that precede the co-penetration of the genitals. It is a time to enjoy the feeling of being desired, savouring these exquisite moments of attentiveness and fine-tuning so that a creative duet can emerge. A man's desire is usually brought to life by gazing at a woman and by the listening ear she lends. A woman needs words that open her heart first, which then connects to her genitals. That is why women are said to be more sentimental.

We have noted that a man's sexuality comes forth from the root of his genitals, while a woman's opens in her heart, on a level with her breasts. Foreplay brings her energies downwards from her heart towards her genitals, while for the man the opposite movement occurs, transferring his energies upwards from his genitals to his heart. So it is the woman's desire touches a man's heart and connects it to his genitals, and the man's words, subtly synchronized with kisses and caresses, move a woman's desire down into her genitals. This process of warming up and adjustment of the senses lights a flame inside a woman that she feels, little by little, inside her pelvis, where it creates the desire to be penetrated.

In this art of the amorous dance, a man and woman stimulate each other by communicating with all their sensory organs. Kisses and caresses open the doors of the erogenous zones: the mouth, the breasts, the clitoris, the penis, the testicles and the entire surface of the skin. Lovers linger over the external surface of the body so that, little by little, they can cross the threshold from external to internal, entwining their tongues as they kiss or using their fingers and their lips on the orifices that open into the body. Each partner gives and abandons while enfolded in the other's arms.

Embracing takes the lovers beyond the boundaries of their physical bodies, creating a shared space of resonance where they get so close that they feel like one. This shared space harks back to the shared feeding space of an infant with the parents, especially the mother. Thanks to the other, each re-experiences their original baby space and contacts the skin of their babyhood.

This sensory skin—that pertains to the erotic—has been forming since the foetal stage and is then further structured by body-to-body affective, energetic and spiritual exchanges, above all with the mother and father. It revives a sensitive, subverbal form of communication experienced before the age of three, in which what we feel or think is also felt by the other. That is why, in love, we no longer need words to understand one another. The other's desire stimulates one's own because the benefits of caresses and kisses come from the intention carried by the vibration of the person performing them. Feeling this intention enables you to abandon yourself to your lover.

Kissing calls on the tongue and the mouth, which is the orifice that, after the navel, is the first life-giving centre at birth, through which we discovered the world and therefore where we experienced our first satisfaction. So, by re-experiencing the sensation of the first organ that penetrated the body, our mother's nipple, we re-experience the confidence that lets us abandon ourself to our lover—or the rigidity and disgust that makes us push him away. If early difficulties prevent an infant from feeding confidently, with gentleness, he or she may later have trouble kissing or accepting a lover's tongue in his/her mouth. Kissing involves an energetic vibration that resonates within the genitals.

The energetic link between the mouth and the genitals is constructed during the foetal period by swallowing amniotic fluid and expelling it from the urinary tract inside the mother's womb. That is why, in lovemaking, the mixing of saliva and the contact of tongues, —"deep kissing"—, is felt in the genitals, recalling the pleasures both of nursing and of swallowing amniotic fluid.

Kissing rekindles all the memories of the love bonds that tied us to our mothers in infancy. When they kiss, a man and woman together experience vibrations like those they each separately experienced with their mother when they were babies. That is a reason why women and men whose emotional life with their mother was difficult in infancy often dislike or are uncomfortable with kissing.

Kisses and caresses can even be aggressive, as if love brings out deficiencies or abuse experienced earlier in life. This produces men and women who cannot have foreplay. They live their sexuality such that their genitals immediately take over, making them feel in charge of their personal creation. For others, foreplay can last "a lifetime." These tend to be women, who were adequately cuddled and loved but were also programmed to remain babies forever. A woman like this can easily achieve the state of bliss she knew as a baby with a man, particularly if she does not know there is anything else to discover.

Fondling the breasts

When aroused by caresses or by the mouth, breasts are a powerful erogenous zone. They grow firm, the nipples get hard, and pleasure goes straight to the genitals. Eroticizing the breasts recalls the pleasure of breastfeeding, during which mother and child occupy the same vibratory space. When a mother's nipples are sucked, it resonates in her uterus, and if the nursing baby is a boy, he may have an erection. So, there is every reason to believe that a baby girl's uterus resonates with her mother's uterus. This explains why a man can be aroused by fondling a woman's breasts. It takes him back not only to the pleasure of touching the breast but also the resonance that he felt in his genitals when he was a nursing baby. But the value of these caresses is erotic: if he sucks the woman's nipple as if he were drinking milk, he is confusing the nutritive and the energetic functions, which may "turn off" the woman. Likewise, Martine realized that she sucked her lover's penis as if she was sucking her mother's breast.

We can see how important it is to recognize what one does not know and to learn to talk about it. Lovers teach each other about the organs whose function they are not acquainted with, creating the shared vibratory space of the amorous encounter.

Fixation on the clitoris

A woman who is not formed to feel the desire to be penetrated, yet confident enough to let herself go, will behave passively just as she did when she was a baby. Her baby girl's body loves her man and lets him love her in the same way she loved her parents and let them love her. Abandoning herself to her man, she may also compensate for what she lacked as a baby and make up for what was missing in infancy. If her man takes her by the hand, takes her in his arms, touches her, caresses her or kisses her, this in itself causes such happiness that she feels self-love: she feels loved and desired. She confidently lets him carry on.

Touching and kissing will eroticize all of her skin, her lips, her breasts, her vulva and her clitoris. The energies of her heart go down to her genitals, and she "gets wet." If her clitoris is stimulated, she will be able to have a clitoral orgasm, harmonizing the sexual energies from her construction as a baby girl. She is satisfied, feels restored and reunified. Very often, for her the duet ends here.

She let this man take her to her own "nirvana" and feels no desire to experience anything else with him. Her voyage is complete, and she withdraws from the erotic exchange. She waits, passive and consenting (in the best case), for her man to finish his monologue on his own, whereas he thought he would continue to share with this woman, who was so well prepared to receive him.

Such a woman reconstitutes herself as a girl, but not as a woman: she has not felt the desire to be penetrated. She has promised her man an encounter which has been cut short, stopping him from reconstituting himself. She confuses the passive and dependent behaviour of being attached inside a mother, or endobiosis (1), with adult sexuality, in which each partner gives and receives to create an active symbiosis.

Desired, but also desiring

Up until this point, a woman has caressed her man's neck, his head, his hair, his torso, his shoulders or his abdomen, but she has not gone as far as his genitals. She has caressed her man as she was caressed when she was small, or as she would like to be caressed, but she has not yet moved on to the pleasure of discovering him sexually.

Feeling desired during foreplay is only part of the adventure. Making love with a man does not stop with the rediscovery of the joys of babyhood—a man is not needed, nor do two genitals need to meet, to achieve those feelings. When a woman is constructed to experience her adult sexuality, foreplay is not just for rediscovering the joys of babyhood and of her sensory skin. It is also, most importantly, to prepare for genitals to fit into each other for the voyage of internal discovery. There is no need to leave the baby's confidence behind but simply to grow up into a sexual adult. In foreplay, all this body language prefigures penetration: we say the two bodies fit together.

A woman then desires the genitals of her man just as much as he desires her and her genitals. She tells him by showing she appreciates this appendage, so different from any part of her own body. She gets to know it, taking pleasure in looking at it, caressing it, honouring it and discovering how it works. It does her good to lavish caresses and kisses upon it. They resonate in her own genitals, strengthening her desire to be penetrated. This appreciation should by no means be seen as a duty she must perform to please him. If so, the doors of sensation have not opened.

Each partner needs to be confirmed by the other's desire, because that is what enables their energies to be in tune. If a woman is incapable of showing appreciation for the man's genitals by fondling his testicles and by feeling the power of his erection inside her mouth, or if the man's genitals disgust

119

her, it is because she was never taught. Her mother never said a word to enable her to see herself as a woman in relation to a man's genitals. It is as if she were the product purely of her mother's womb, as if her father had nothing to do with her presence in the world. If as a child she was unable to create an image of adult sexuality, she cannot conceive of it as being an occasion for sharing, for difference and complementarity between men and women.

For a man, a woman's desire for his genitals is essential to his well-being and gives him the energy he needs to continue on the erotic journey with her. The desire to discover and to stimulate the woman's genitals—to know how they work by kissing them with his mouth and his tongue—takes him back to his origins, as Gustave Courbet so beautifully captured in a painting by calling it *The Origin of the World*. The warmth, softness, scents and tastes that make up the landscape in which a man immerses himself further increase his desire for her. When she knows in turn how to express the pleasure he is giving her, foreplay becomes more intense for him and defers his haste to penetrate her.

If she feels apprehensive, though, her partner will sense it. It's true that a level of inner security and confidence is needed in order to feel the desire to make love. As Marjorie put it, "It only goes well when I feel secure, and there are still times when I don't. It's an essential precondition for me now. I've learned that if I don't feel secure, I can't let myself go." Marjorie is grateful that she pleases her man, but she doesn't feel the desire to make love with him. She wants to want him, but her heart is not in it: it is not sufficiently "empty," as the ancient Chinese said (2)—that is, not sufficiently available for desire. Such a woman feels as if she were cut in two. Unable to be present to herself, she cannot be present to someone else.

This is why, if the love experienced in a woman's childhood was incoherent—invasive, overwhelming and suffocating, or on the other hand insufficient and lacking—she finds it hard to let

120

herself be caressed and kissed and even harder to be penetrated: she lacks confidence in her partner. "My mother drew me towards her and hugged me so hard that I literally suffocated. My attempts to back away just made her embrace stronger. So, I learned to keep absolutely still, to feel nothing, to clench my jaw, stiffen my shoulders and wait until she was willing to disengage" (3).

When a man takes this sort of woman in his arms, she may once again fear being held prisoner, which prevents her from opening herself to him. Her fear that love will turn into confinement comes from her mother's devouring love. Other women, on the contrary, will unconsciously reproduce their mother's devouring love with their man. They do not realize that their love is stifling him, that for him it is an undercurrent that will drag him down. These women do not understand that such love destroys the man's erotic desire and sometimes makes him run away.

Benefitting from what we do not have

Although love implies reuniting with a known infantile state, its aim is to make us curious to discover something new and to welcome the unknown. Through penetration, the genitals exchange their vibratory powers so that both partners benefit from what they do not have. Therefore, making love is a celebration, a kind of magic that arises from coming alive together due to difference and complementarity. It helps us reconstitute and strengthen ourselves.

For women who are described or who describe themselves as "clitoral," the problem is not that they have a clitoral orgasm, but rather that they think clitoral orgasm sufficient for sexual encounter. To feel the life-force of one's genitals inside one's body there has to be exchange, a greater, more subtle and complete agreement.

A clitoral orgasm is just the beginning of a process which should naturally make us want to go further, to discover an interior and an elsewhere that are otherwise not ours. Reaching out for this elsewhere involves wanting the genitals to come alive, allowing them to open to sensation, and conceptualizing penetration as the possibility that the genitals of two partners can, through their encounter, come alive together.

At each stage of lovemaking, with each new exploration, inhibitions may appear. These always take us back to our own history. Contrary to what we may want to believe, these obstructions are rarely our partner's fault. It is wiser and more effective to proceed from the assumption that coming together with someone else is awakening a personal issue of one's own. Unknown until just now, this issue established itself with our parents but could not be resolved by them. In this sense, love is what opens our eyes to the wounds from the past, allowing us to come to terms with them and heal them.

A woman who does not find within herself the desire to be penetrated but lets herself be carried along just so she can respond to her man's desire, is offering him something that cannot fully satisfy him. But above all she is depriving herself of the regenerative pleasure which, according to Chinese medicine, has the power to keep illness away.

The co-penetration of the genitals

Love is revitalizing and thus therapeutic if the co-penetration of the genitals is at once physical, energetic, emotional and psychological. When a woman feels her vagina vibrate in contact with a man's penis, she feels this vibration as another life inside her, which she welcomes and loves and vitalizes. This ability to welcome inside her body one of the most alive parts of a man prefigures what will happen when she is expecting a child. It is a fundamental experience that will help her to lead a more complete life overall, and also to welcome that child.

Creating the phallus

A man penetrates, a woman welcomes. Their sexes fit into each other to create a new, shared vibratory space which each of them nourishes by giving more and more to the other and by receiving more and more from the other.

The encounter of the feminine and the masculine elements of two partners in erotic climax makes them together and mutually more dynamic, more complete, more fully empowered. The difference between the sexes exists only in our physical body, beyond which we are all bisexual. In ancient China, sexual pleasure was said to come from the union of the masculine principle, Yang, and the feminine principle, Yin. But since one never exists without the other, the masculine and the feminine coexist in each of us.

The complementarity of the genitals can no longer be seen as a matter of penetrating or being penetrated. It is mutual co-penetration, established by the vibratory contact of the mucous membranes. In a vibratory duet, the genitals exchange. They speak to each other and dance together. The phallus is not just a man's penis or a solitary erection, as it is often misleadingly depicted. It is a masculine amalgam created by two partners and is also constituted by the female genitals into which it fits. Each partner's genitals nourish the phallus with their own energy to procure pleasure for the man and the woman.

Feeling the uterus and maintaining the fire

A woman psychically connects with a man's sexual forces, which come from his testicles, to receive them in her uterus. In terms of sexual energy, the uterus becomes the resonance chamber and the alchemical crucible for the meeting of the masculine and feminine sexual forces, the Yin and the Yang, the Water and the Fire of each partner.

From the uterus, pleasure can spread fully throughout the inside of each body, not just the woman's, but also the man's. For him, it is an invitation to penetrate with all his energies.

When pleasure is vaginal, a woman receives the power of the masculine genitals, which regenerates and consolidates her, but she nonetheless goes no further than the vestibule. It is the uterus that serves as the centre from where the breaths of their sexual joy can expand throughout the body.

For a woman, feeling the power of this energy is the revelation of her femininity, the living proof of her body's creative power. It is a "celestial elevator" that carries her energy upwards to the top of her body and even beyond, connecting her to the skies. Thus, the man, the "bearer of Heaven" as the Chinese tradition says, roots himself in a woman's genitals and replenishes his energy there. If a woman does not welcome his sexual energies, a man cannot contact the source and achieve full satisfaction. In this exchange, a woman's role is to "tend the fire" that supports a man's erection. It is by receiving the fire of his sexual energy and expressing how she is vibrating with the feeling of its power, that she tends that fire.

Sometimes a man loses his erection at the moment of penetration, even though he ardently desires the woman. Contrary to common belief, the man is not the only one responsible. The woman has an important role in sustaining his erection. If she has not created the necessary space within herself to welcome his sex, or if she does not know how to tend his fire, a man can lose his erection and so lose his bearings. A man can also lose his erection because of the intensity of his love for his woman, which, in the midst of lovemaking, may cause him to unconsciously confuse her body with the body of his mother. This happens fairly often when the man becomes a father or when he makes a commitment out of deep love.

In lovemaking, each partner reveals the other's pleasures, but also their difficulties, by taking them both back to their respective family and individual histories.

Being fully present to oneself and to the other at the same time

At this stage, it is important to be wholly present, both to yourself and to the other. The fact of having created a shared vibratory space makes this possible: the two of you are in a state of empathy. To achieve this requires complete availability for the exchange and so it is worth setting aside time to do this so as to be clear about the objective of your coming together.

When making love, as soon as one of the two is distracted by an intruding thought, getting lost either within oneself or elsewhere, becoming absent, the energetic body the two make up deflates like a balloon. Communication is broken and is felt by the other to be a brutal decline in energy. The two bodies find themselves in two separate spaces, no longer linked.

Sustaining one's presence both to yourself and to your partner is demanding. When we are so fully with someone else, we risk forgetting ourself being aware only of our partner's energy, without taking into account our own. Conversely, when we are fully present to ourself, we might well forget our partner. You might see yourself alone in your own energetic space with no concern for your partner. You are no longer with him.

Finding words again

To maintain the energetic communication, it is time for words again. To genuinely express what we feel, to be able to say what is happening in us by describing images or sensations, to say how we perceive our partner, to show him how his body turns us on—this is a way of keeping connected and of sustaining each other's creativity.

During foreplay, you find yourself in a subverbal world. You are cut off from words. Verbal expression, if it exists, is like baby talk: "my sweetie," "my darling." It brings back old memories.

Its function has more to do with energy than with meaning. These utterances are aimed at enhancing pleasure.

Now, as we have seen, the baby has grown up. Finding speech again allows lovers to stay in communication, to know where the other stands. We might say that orgasm is a matter of energy, while a love that grows deeper is a matter of words. Without speech, an erotic relationship cannot be built. Nor can it take root over time. "Love without words, it's as if I were alone, closed off in my shell," as a colleague at a workshop on sexuality put it. Speech creates the confidence needed to open yourself to your partner. It allows sexual energy to take the path best suited to the particular circumstances.

At each turn in the road, erotic communication may encounter an obstacle. It is important to consider the obstacles within yourself, since they interfere with communication. One can go on making love, but the amorous exchange may be halted by the same issue over and again without our being able to move beyond. These obstacles hinder further fulfilment. Removing them opens up new places to explore.

It is important for partners to speak to each other and to take stock of the situation while keeping in mind that one partner cannot be expected to solve the other's problems and vice-versa. Some problems must be resolved on one's own account with the help of a therapist, so as not to burden one's partner nor ask him for the impossible. If each accepts responsibility for personal problems, and for doing something about them, the dialogue can become creative again.

Pathways of sexual energy

Sexual energy is bigger than we are. We need to let it circulate. The energy may rise throughout, as if our skin was the surface of a container that fills from bottom to top. Or it may nourish our organs—when we are acquainted with them we can feel them getting stronger. Or again, sexual energy takes the particular energetic paths described in manuals on sexual alchemy (4), especially the "little celestial revolution." In this case the energy moves up the spinal column returns down the mid-line on the front of the body, creating a ring that effectively encapsulates the energy of the sexual adult body.

Completeness and surpassing oneself

For everyone, love is an opening into the unknown realm of our life forces, the forces that gave us life. Lovemaking brings these forces into play. It allows us not just to discover ourselves, but to transcend ourselves in an improvised creative duet.

The energies thus awakened begin by invading us. They spread through the abdomen, filling all its organs. They cross the diaphragm, invading the lungs, heart, and throat, and go on to enter the head. They rise to our brain and inundate it. We can see more clearly, hear better, our ideas are sharp. We feel strong, upright, more in harmony with ourselves.

We have reshaped ourselves. This energetic power fertilizes our entire body. It makes us confident and calm. That assurance makes us more secure on our base, where our original garden—the one called secret—now freshly irrigated, breathes anew. Like all gardens, it is cultivated, it flowers, it receives visitors and is tended to differently depending on the season, the time of day, the inspiration of the moment, age and experience.

Projecting oneself into the other's body

In love, because two bodies become one, our mind has the power to project itself into a part of our lover's body. We need only concentrate mentally on a part for him to feel that part growing stronger.

This practice allows lovers to explore each other. It is common knowledge that a man can enter a woman with his energies. There is less awareness that a woman can do the same: the psychological dimension of her masculine energy enables her to mentally project herself into a man's body, making it possible for their coming together to last longer by supplying him with energy.

Jouissance: sexual joy

Sexual joy (*jouissance*) is not just an act; it is a process which is sensed and mastered. It is a phenomenon that is studied in wave physics under the term "resonance." The bodies' pleasure from co-penetration comes from the energies brought into play by the two partners, who seek to enter into resonance: to vibrate in unison, at the same frequency. It is like singing a duet, when two voices harmonize and potentiate each other's power, becoming one voice.

The partners' bodies feel light. They are in "seventh heaven."

A man and a woman bring each other to orgasm, and it is important not to fixate on the idea of reaching orgasm at the same instant. Love must remain open to one's own creativity as much as to that of one's partner. It is a musical score for two, and the instruments take turns, as in an orchestra. Each time we make love, the harmonics change according to each partner's readiness and depending on our time of life. The waves that are called into play are not always the same in quantity and quality each time we make love. These differences are even more apparent between different partners.

We also need to get rid of false, preconceived ideas, which categorize, judge and paralyze a sexual relationship. We have to stop thinking there are men who are permanently impotent or habitual premature ejaculators; or women who are irredeemably frigid or definitively clitoral. We need to keep in mind that sexuality is an open system where everything hinges on the quality of the relationship established.

What matters is the place we attribute to our sexuality in our lives: setting aside time, energy and words; giving it as much consideration as we give to work, to children, to anything that matters to us. If we let down our guard, the old structures will catch up with us, and gain the upper hand. They will absorb all our energy so that we neglect the feminine sexual part of ourselves.

What is an orgasm?

Orgasm is the culminating point of resonance of all the forces at play when making love. To reach orgasm, it helps to have confidence in the vibratory phenomena, to be unafraid of losing control of what is happening. Suddenly, there's a leap or a plunge that requires you to open yourself to it and go with it. For a woman, orgasm means feeling that a man has plunged his penis inside her and that she is carried by him. For a man, orgasmic pleasure is additionally sensing how his energy invades a woman's body and feeling responsible for the luminous uplift that comes from the union of their two energetic bodies.

A woman's orgasm involves many layers that unfold simultaneously. It is the physical sensation of vibratory waves that start in the vagina and spread at various speeds through the body. At the same time, it is an emotional sensation that comes from ideas and thoughts: "I feel the energetic force of the man who penetrates my body," said a colleague in a workshop. "It's as if a door suddenly opens to let him inside me. For several moments, my body is weightless and out of my control. For me, the real pleasure of orgasm is in this sensation of rising, created by this wave that spreads everywhere. The wave begins in my belly and bursts in my head going out through my eyes, my mouth, and the top of my skull. It makes me feel connected to the sky."

"Orgasm," another colleague said, "is a moment of intense pleasure, which comes from my sexual organs and the voluptuous warmth of the belly and goes on to intensely enfold my whole body. Like magic, the climax gradually tiptoes in then suddenly takes us off at a gallop. Then it subsides, followed by a state of deep satisfaction, leaving me fulfilled and content."

"There are also magical moments when orgasmic pleasure gushes forth without warning," said a third. "Abruptly, with a caress, or with the sweetness of penetration, I can feel my genitals. They swell and go into a series of spasms that develop by steps and spread through my whole body. I am plunged into a universe of vibrations, images, and colours. I become a shoreline stroked by the waves of the high seas. They roll over me, big or small, but their slightest touch floods the secret recesses of my body with rapturous sensations. Behind my closed eyes, a dazzling blue carries me into a world of light."

Attaining such ecstatic states requires true presence. They are made possible by both partners being in an affective and emotional state such that they feel fully supportive of and receptive to the other, totally confident both in their own forces and in those of their partner.

This account expresses the discovery of sexual joy through the subjectivity of a woman:

> "Learning to make love has been rapturous. It makes me feel the way I want to feel. It's a revelation and a crystallization of myself. I still can't believe that the meeting of bodies can create such feelings; that my genitals are a gateway to a wonderland; that they are yearned for as such brings me great happiness. My self-esteem grows, I feel proud and, my femininity is confirmed—something I have always wanted. I feel structured, whole, upright, alive, clear and most of all relieved of my psychological phantoms. Coming together with a partner contributes to my self-respect.
>
> Jouissance means to vibrate, to be active and responsive to the sensations this man provokes in me: a man who I like and who likes me. I feel his penis in me, his

penis in me gives me pleasure. Both like a victory and something inexorable. I let life find a home inside my body. How this man's organ brings a thrust from eternity which takes us back there! Our two genitals are the intermediaries for the discovery of new dimensions.

Now I know how to tell a man I like that I want him. I use my erotic vocabulary to describe the trip we will take, how I am the host and he is the virile power.

I tell him and show him how he is in his rightful place when he is inside my body, how much I love it, how his masculine power moves through me. I tell him what I am experiencing by way of sensations and images. So, off we go. We depart on our voyage. He is on horseback and I am the horse who leads him through my garden, its magnificent alleys, groves and scents. I love the kisses of our mouths and his caresses of my breasts that make my genitals come alive. Another time the horse becomes Pegasus, and I take off into the cosmos, propelled by our genitals fitting together. I can also find myself in the depths of the seas, propelled forward by a small rocket. Sometimes I am the rider, proud and dignified who, with age, has lost fire but gained depth. The more I give myself to him, the more I feel him within myself. Now I can project myself into his body. That is when the sensations take over. Mentally, I let my intuition take me into his organs or his energy circuits, and I tell him what is happening.

And when I sense that he is about to ejaculate, I back off ever so slightly, to create a pause, to bring down the intensity so it can come back with renewed force.

Power concentrates in the genitals and rises to the orifices of the face. It gathers strength. The vibrations intensify up to the paroxysm where, suspended in time, his ejaculation brings completion to this coming together.

Coming down after making love

"It was an unforgettable night, not because of the erotic details but because of the joy of feeling myself whole, without being torn between my sexual impulses and my deepest feelings."

At the end of this trip, cosmic or otherwise, lovers feel reconstituted and more complete. They have known each other, in the biblical sense. They are regenerated and they feel empowered. They marvel at what they have just experienced and each feels gratitude towards the other, wanting to offer thanks and loving the other even more. The man and woman have thus put into effect the marvellous alchemy of the senses. In terms of the ancient Chinese texts, they have just "gathered the remedy that protects against illness." Such a benefit becomes imprinted in the body's memory and makes them want to repeat it.

To celebrate coming together in carnal knowledge is to honour life. Any celebration of life does us good; it lets us approach its mystery. This exchange brings into play creative forces which previously gave us life and now belong to us. We make them even stronger when, by offering them to the other, we receive theirs. Knowing how to gather these forces gives us an energy that steadies us on our feet, straightens us up and propels us into our human reality.

Notes

1. See Jean-Louis Revardel, *Constance et fantaisie du vivant* (Paris: Albin Michel, 1993).
2. See Claude Larre, Élisabeth Rochat de la Vallée, *Les mouvements du coeur. Psychologie des Chinoises.* Paris: Desclée de Brouwer, 1992. Translated as *Rooted in Spirit: The Heart of Chinese Medicine* (Station Hill Press, 1995).
3. Chitra Banerjee Divakaruni, *Arranged Marriage: Stories* (Random House, 1997).
4. See Catherine Despeux, *Immortelles de la Chine ancienne* (Paris: Pardès, 1997); Mantak Chia, *Healing Love*, *op. cit.*

ACKNOWLEDGEMENT

Fifteen years after the first French publication, I continue to be flattered by the unexpected popularity of this book and am deeply grateful to see it now available to anglophone readers. If it can help some develop a better understanding of the workings of sexuality within their relationship with their partner and move a few steps forward towards a healthier family and greater self-fulfillment, my book will have attained its goal.

This English edition never would have existed without Wendy Hollway's steadfast belief in the need for a translation; she was instrumental in convincing the publisher of its importance. Furthermore, her scholarly background as a professor of psychology, coupled with interests in transgenerational psychoanalysis and Chinese medicine, made her the ideal candidate to take on the translation. I am thankful to have met her.

I would also like to give credit to Maxine Weaver for her early translation, Virginia Popper for her generous and ingenious collaboration to clarify some abstruse concepts and make them more accessible to the English reader, and Divya Kumar-Dumas who worked closely with me to ensure the fidelity of this English translation to my original prose.

I continue to be grateful to many people who helped bring the first French edition to life: Didier Dumas, with whom I elaborated and developed much of this research, who was my travelling companion in life and the father of my children; Patricia Canino, whose assistance and generous collaboration provided the clarity necessary to write the original version of this book; Christophe Guias, editing director at Payot for his unwavering support; all my clients with whom I travelled this road of discovery; many participants in research groups on generational transmission at the Jardin d'Idées; and the innumerable friends, young and not so young, who supported me in myriad ways along the way.

INDEX

acute ailments, 29–31. *See also*
  recurrent disorders
adult love, 6
affective encoding, 52. *See also*
  sexual construction
  of girls
affective touching between father
  and child, 47. *See also*
  sexual construction
  of girls
after-pains, 51
age of reason, 62
ailments. *See also* recurrent
  disorders
 acute, 29–31
 gynaecological, 83–85
ancestral memory, 88–89.
    See also gynaecological
  family tree
anniversary syndrome, 85
art of the bedchamber, 11–12.
    See also sexual anatomy
aversion to maternal function, 80

bedchamber, art of, 11–12
birth control, 97–98

breast, 23. *See also* sexual anatomy
 -feeding, 23, 50–52
 fondling, 117. *See also*
  making love

caresses, 113–117. *See also*
  making love
carnal communication, 13
cervix, 17–18. *See also* sexual
  anatomy
child, unplanned, 98
Chinese medicine, 36–37. *See also*
  sexual anatomy
 perverse energy, 93, 94
 principle of, 12
 vital breath, 36–37
Chinese sexology, x. *See also*
  Chinese medicine
 art of the bedchamber, 11–12
clitoral orgasm, 15, 121–122.
    See also making love
clitoris, 14–16. *See also* sexual
  anatomy
 fixation on, 118
closed adoption, 74
communication, carnal, 13

135

compenetrate, 27
contraceptive pills, 85, 97–98
co-penetration, 27. *See also*
        making love
    of genitals, 122
courtship displays, 114. *See also*
        making love
cystitis, 10, 26, 42. *See also*
        recurrent disorders;
        sexual anatomy

desire, 112. *See also* making love;
        sexual desire
    desired and desiring, 119–121
    third, 24
disorders, 40. *See also* recurrent
        disorders
Dolto, F., xi, xiii, xvi
duplication, 91
dyad stage, 55–57. *See also* sexual
        construction of girls

encoding, affective, 52. *See also*
        sexual construction
        of girls
engrams, 22, 43, 56. *See also*
        recurrent disorders;
        sexual anatomy
erogenous zones, 115. *See also*
        making love

falling in love. *See* love, falling in
fallopian tubes, 18. *See also* sexual
        anatomy
fathering, 41
father's role and difference
        between sexes, 60–64.
        See also sexual
        construction of girls
female sexuality, 35
feminine dynamic, xiv

fondling the breasts, 117. *See also*
        making love
foreplay, 114–117. *See also*
        making love
freeze-frame, 84. *See also*
        gynaecological
        family tree
functional problem, 94

genealogy, 87–89. *See also*
        gynaecological
        family tree
genital, 40. *See also* recurrent
        disorders
    awareness, 50
    co-penetration of, 122
    educating about, 64–65
    encounter between, 114–117
genosociogram, 89–92. *See also*
        gynaecological
        family tree
GREEN, 46–47, 74
gynaecological
    ailments, 83–85
    disorders, 81
    symptoms, 85
gynaecological family tree, 75
    ancestral memory, 88–89
    anniversary syndrome, 85
    aversion to maternal
        function, 80
    care, 92–94
    contraceptive pills, 85
    duplication, 91
    freeze-frame, 84
    functional problem, 94
    genealogy, 87–89
    genosociogram, 89–92
    gynaecological ailments and
        origins, 83–85
    gynaecological disorders, 81

gynaecological symptoms, 85
organic problem, 94
painful menstruation, 75–81
perverse energy, 93, 94
phantom disorders, 81
premenstrual syndrome, 82–83
repetition, 84–85
repetitive phenomena, 91
sterility and infertility, 86
symptoms generated by
family line disorders,
85–86
unwanted pregnancies, 86–87

haptonomy, 46, 100
hormonal control, 19–20. *See also*
sexual anatomy
hymen, 16–17. *See also* sexual
anatomy

incest, 63
incestuous energy bond,
47–48. *See also* sexual
construction of girls
infertility, 86
inherited social and cultural
burdens, 96–97. *See also*
sexual desire
inhibitions, 122
invaginated, 105–106, 107. *See also*
sexual desire

jouissance, xv, xvi–xvii, 128–129.
See also making love

kissing, 116–117

latency period, 68
life force inhabiting us, 42–43.
See also recurrent
disorders

love, adult, 6
love, falling in, 1
adult love, 6
first object of love, 2
infantile eroticism, 4
loving like child, 2–3
loving men like loving
mothers, 1–2
maternal love, 6–8
mother–child dyad, 8
regression, 6
woman and mother in us, 4–5
lovemaking. *See* making love

making love, 38–40, 113. *See also*
recurrent disorders
being fully present, 125
caresses, 113–117
clitoral orgasm, 121–122
coming down after, 132
completeness and surpassing
oneself, 127
co-penetration of genitals, 122
courtship displays, 114
creating the phallus, 123
desired and desiring, 119–121
erogenous zones, 115
feeling uterus and maintaining
fire, 123–124
fixation on clitoris, 118
fondling the breasts, 117
foreplay and encounter
between genitals,
114–117
inhibitions, 122
jouissance, 128–129
kissing, 116–117
orgasm, 129–131
projecting oneself into other's
body, 127–128
resonance, 128

sensory skin, 115–116
sexual energy pathways,
    126–127
shared space, 115
verbal expression, 125–126
for women, xii
maternal function, aversion to, 80
maternal love, 6–8
matrix, original, 41. *See also*
    recurrent disorders
memory, ancestral, 88–89. *See also*
    gynaecological
    family tree
menstruation, 75–81. *See also*
    gynaecological
    family tree
mother
    –child dyad, 8
    death of, 68–72. *See also*
        sexual construction
        of girls
motherhood training
    department, 53
mothering, 41

names and surnames, 48–50

Oedipal phase, 57
    end of, 62
oophoritis, 42. *See also* recurrent
    disorders
organic problem, 94
orgasm, xvii, 129–131. *See also*
    making love
    clitoral, 121–122
    types, 15
original matrix, 41. *See also*
    recurrent disorders
origination
    phase of. *See* dyad stage
    theory of, 43

ovaries, 18–19. *See also* sexual
    anatomy

parental. *See also* sexual
    construction of girls
    fulfillment, 100
    intimacy, 65–66
pelvic floor. *See* perineum
pelvis, 20. *See also* sexual anatomy
penetration, 104. *See also*
    sexual desire
perineum, 9, 21–23. *See also* sexual
    anatomy
perverse energy, 93, 94
phallus, 123. *See also* making love
phantom disorders, 81. *See also*
    gynaecological
    family tree
pituitary gland, 20
pregnancies, unwanted, 86–87
premenstrual syndrome, 82–83
projecting oneself into other's
    body, 127–128. *See also*
    making love
psychologically pregnant, 51–52
pyelonephritis, 42. *See also*
    recurrent disorders

questioning phase, 67–68

recurrent ailments, 29–31. *See also*
    recurrent disorders
recurrent disorders, 29, 30
    acute ailments, 29–31
    blocked sexuality, 33–36
    Chinese medicine, 36–37
    disrupting repetition, 37–38
    engrams, 43
    inhabiting life force, 42–43
    looking for origin, 31–33
    making love, 38–40

mothering, 41
original matrix, 41
recurrent ailments, 29–31
sexual desire, 37
teaching genitals, 40–42
theory of origination, 43
thrush infection, 30
regression, 6
repetition, 84–85, 91. *See also*
    gynaecological
    family tree
resonance, 128

salpingitis, 42. *See also* recurrent
    disorders
self-recognition, 59–60. *See also*
    sexual construction
    of girls
sensory awareness, 107
sensory skin, 115–116
sexual
    arousal, 9
    desire, 12
    energy, 9–12, 25–26
    gynaecology, 105
    joy. See *jouissance*
    liberation, 98–100
    openness, xv
    pleasure and uterus, 13–14
    system, 19–20
sexual anatomy, 9
    art of the bedchamber, 11–12
    breasts and breastfeeding, 23
    carnal communication, 13
    cervix, 17–18
    changes in woman's body,
        23–25
    Chinese medicine principle, 12
    clitoris, 14–16
    cystitis and sexual energy, 10
    engrams, 22

fallopian tubes, 18
hormonal control, 19–20
hymen, 16–17
orgasm types, 15
ovaries, 18–19
pelvis, 20
perineum, 9, 21–23
sexual arousal, 9
sexual desire, 12
sexual energy, 9–12, 25–26
sexual system life cycle, 19–20
symphyses, 21
uterus, 13–14, 17–18
vagina, 17
vulva, 14
sexual construction of girls, 45
    affective encoding from
        parents, 52
    affective touching in father
        and child, 47
    after-pains, 51
    breast-feeding, 50–52
    building girl's sexuality, 52–55
    dyad stage, 55–57
    educating about genitals,
        64–65
    end of Oedipal phase, 62
    engrams, 56
    expecting little girl, 45–47
    falling into depression, 68–72
    father's role and difference
        between sexes, 60–64
    haptonomy, 46
    incest, 63
    incestuous energy bond, 47–48
    to know about conception,
        57–59
    latency period, 68
    meaning and renewal, 72–74
    motherhood training
        department, 53

mother's death, 68–72
names and surnames, 48–50
Oedipal phase, 57
parental intimacy, 65–66
parents as models, 54
psychologically pregnant,
    51–52
questioning phase, 67–68
self-recognition, 59–60
sex and death, 67–68
sexuality, celebrating, 57
sexuality in family
    atmosphere, 66
split sexuality, 65
transgenerational
    phantoms, 55
unfrigid woman, 56
sexual construction of woman,
    link affecting, 35
sexual desire, 12, 37, 95, 112.
        See also recurrent
        disorders; sexual
        anatomy
    birth control, 97–98
    breaking transgenerational
        repetition, 106–109
    continued ignorance about
        sexuality, 100–101
    dissatisfaction, 105
    expressing, 101–102
    floating heads, 111
    inherited social and cultural
        burdens, 96–97
    inhibition, 102–105
    invaginated, 105–106, 107
    in man and women, 109–111
    parental fulfillment, 100
    penetration, 104
    radical upheaval, 97
    sensory awareness, 107

sexual gynaecology, 105
sexual liberation, 98–100
sexual energy. *See also* sexual
        anatomy
    circulation, 9–12. *See also*
        sexual anatomy
    cystitis and, 10
    in motion, 25–26
    pathways, 126–127. *See also*
        making love
sexuality, xi, xii, 53. *See also*
        sexual construction
        of girls
    blocked, 33–36
    in family atmosphere, 66
    female, 35
    ignorance about, 100–101
    into one's life, xiii
    of pleasure, xiv
    revitalizing, xvi
shared space, 115
split sexuality, 65
sterility, 86
symphyses, 21. *See also* sexual
        anatomy

Taoism, 12
theory of origination, 43.
        See also recurrent
        disorders
third desire, 24
thrush, 42. *See also* recurrent
        disorders
TONG, 27
touching between father and
        child, affective, 47
transgenerational phantoms, 55
transgenerational repetition,
        106–109. *See also*
        sexual desire

unfrigid woman, 56
unplanned child, 98
unwanted pregnancies, 86–87
uterine body, 18
uterus, 13–14, 17–18. *See also*
        sexual anatomy

vagina, 17. *See also* sexual anatomy
vaginal orgasm, 15
vaginitis, 42. *See also* recurrent
        disorders
verbal expression, 125–126.
        See also making love

vital breath (*Qi*), 36–37
vulva, 14. *See also* sexual anatomy
vulvitis, 42. *See also* recurrent
        disorders

Western medicine, 30
woman's body, changes in, 23–25.
        See also sexual anatomy
woman's sexual construction, link
        affecting, 35

Yin Yang, 26